ALLERGIES AND INFECTIOUS DISEASES

CAMPYLOBACTER INFECTIONS

EPIDEMIOLOGY, CLINICAL MANAGEMENT AND PREVENTION

ALLERGIES AND INFECTIOUS DISEASES

Additional books in this series can be found on Nova's website under the Series tab.

Additional e-books in this series can be found on Nova's website under the e-book tab.

ALLERGIES AND INFECTIOUS DISEASES

CAMPYLOBACTER INFECTIONS

EPIDEMIOLOGY, CLINICAL MANAGEMENT AND PREVENTION

BRITTANY A. BERTUCCI
EDITOR

NOVA BIOMEDICAL

New York

Library of Congress Cataloging-in-Publication Data

ISBN: 978-1-63463-858-6
Library of Congress Control Number: 2014959219

Published by Nova Science Publishers, Inc. † New York

Contents

Preface

This book discusses the epidemiology, clinical management and prevention of *Campylobacter* infections.

Chapter 1 – *Campylobacter jejuni* is the leading cause of bacterial enteritis in the world and this zoonotic disease is mainly transmitted by food and water. *Campylobacter* infections are characterized by several symptoms such as watery/bloody diarrhea, abdominal pain, fever, headache, nausea and vomiting, which may persist for a few days. Post-infection complications are also observed, principally neurological disorders (Guillain-Barré syndrome) or reactive arthritis.

Many factors involved in *Campylobacter* virulence have been described in the literature. However, their intervention in the pathogenesis mechanism is still being investigated and their connections with the clinical signs of disease have not been clearly determined. Among the well-characterized virulence factors are flagella, responsible for motility and type III secretion of effectors, and intestinal colonization. In addition to the putative adhesins and invasins, the lipooligosaccharide (LOS) is involved in adhesion to/invasion of host cells and the mimicking of ganglioside sugars. The mechanisms of other virulence factors, such as the Cia proteins (*Campylobacter* invasion antigens) involved in invasion and the type VI secretion system recently described as interacting with the host, are not fully understood. Epidemiological analyses have revealed that the majority of genes encoding for virulence factors are present in the different *C. jejuni* strains, whatever their origin. Some of these genes contain inserted sequences or punctual mutations, which could be used as molecular tools to detect and identify *Campylobacter* spp.. Despite scientific advances concerning *C. jejuni* during the last decade, the knowledge and understanding of the virulence mechanisms of *Campylobacter* need further research. The objective here is to review the consensus virulence factors of *C. jejuni* pathogenesis in order to contribute to the risk management strategies for this foodborne pathogen and identify potential avenues to detect robust virulence factors.

Chapter 2 – *Campylobacter* is now considered as a major agent of bacteriological foodborne diseases. This microorganism is capable to cause a very large number of cases of digestive campylobacteriosis, worldwide. Its high intestinal carriage by several livestock (poultry, swine, bovine, ovine…) is the reason why these animals are primary reservoirs of this microorganism. The quantitative importance of these primary reservoirs leads to its introduction into various habitats and to a contamination of foods, which can take place at any stage of the food production. After contamination, its survival and its ability to cause disease after ingestion of a low minimum infective dose do the rest. The disease is present in all parts of the world, preferably in summer, and in all populations, but with peaks for the age groups 0-5 years, 20-30 years and above 60 years. Medical treatment may be conventional, often symptomatic, sometimes associated with the use of antibiotics in some severe cases. The development of a vaccine strategy is difficult even if there have been significant advances in recent years in the field. However, digestive campylobacteriosis transmitted by foods are not unavoidable because there are, at all stages of the food chain, many truly effective control measures to reduce the contamination of foods by Campylobacter. Their effective implementation and coordination in an integrated approach of hygiene management, will reduce the incidence of this disease.

Chapter 3 – The genus *Campylobacter* comprises Gram-negative spiral-shaped bacteria, which can cause a foodborne illness in humans called campylobacteriosis; the infection generally occurs through the consumption of undercooked chicken or ready-to-eat meals that have been in contact with contamined raw chicken. The occurrence of pathogens in foods may be caused by cross-contamination, mainly due to insufficient hygiene of the staff and the environment, and/or by improper conditions enabling survival and growth of microorganisms, like inadequate cooking or temperature abuse.

In Europe, the general principles and requisites of food safety legislation have been established by Regulation (EC) 178/2002, followed by Regulation (EC) 852/2004 on the hygiene of foodstuffs. One of the basic obligations foreseen by Regulation (EC) 852/2004 is that food businesses operators have to implement permanent procedures based on Hazard Analysis and Critical Control Point (HACCP) principles in order to ensure the safety of products.

In recent years, public catering has taken on an increasingly important role in the lives of working people, and food safety linked to the consumption of out-of-home meals has become a critical issue; in particular, the increase in the cases of campylobacteriosis highlights the need for continuous monitoring and control of the presence of *Campylobacter* spp. in the food chain.

The European Food Safety Authority (EFSA) estimates that the cost of the episodes of campylobacteriosis for the health system, in terms of lost productivity in the European Union, is around € 2.4 billion a year. Recent microbiological studies conducted in the United Kingdom, Ireland, Spain and Denmark showed that cases of *Campylobacter* infection (well recognised or not) depended largely upon an incorrect application of good manufacturing procedures, hygiene related to the handling of raw materials (mainly poulty meat) and cooking. This last procedure was recognised as one of the main critical points. To date, the Commission Decision (EC) 516/2007 regulates the tolerance to the presence of thermotolerant species of *Campylobacter* on slaughtered carcasses, but it does not specify tolerances for foods ready for consumption, as already provided for other pathogens such as *Salmonella* spp. and *Listeria monocytogenes*. Though current European legislation on zoonoses requires prompt notification of episodes of human infectious diseases to the National Health System, a lack of official data occurs in several European Countries because of the absence of harmonized procedures for monitoring and recording the cases of campylobacteriosis.

Chapter 4 – The infection by *Campylobacter* spp. constitutes a worldwide distribution of zoonosis, with serious repercussions for public health and a significant socio-economic impact. Representatives of this genus are the most common etiologic agents of gastroenteritis caused by food. *C. jejuni* and *C. coli* are recognized as the most important species and with greater pathogenic potential from the food safety's point of view. The raw milk consumption, non potable water, and other food of animal origin might be the source of human infection. However, poultry is an important reservoir of *Campylobacter*, thus becomes the main target of control measures. Understanding the epidemiology of *Campylobacter* and the main challenges in its control, contributes to determine the risk posed to human health. The difficulty of isolating and cultivating *Campylobacter;* and the high cost, results in a lack of accurate data in the diseases' occurrence in the world. It is known that despite the apparent *Campylobacter*'s fragility to the environmental conditions, this agent is able to create mechanisms that allow their metabolic adaptation and growth change quickly in different environmental conditions in which they are submitted. This ability allows the detection of different behaviors that can explain their ability to survive and multiply in stressful conditions. These parameters directly affect the prevalence and persistence of *Campylobacter* in food destined for consumption. The epidemiology of infections caused by *Campylobacter* spp. are considered complex, presenting multiple determinants in this microorganism spread. Among these factors, are represented important virulence factors in the agent's pathogenesis, resulting in greater severity of clinical disease. The infection by *Campylobacter* causes gastroenteritis in humans and takes place orally through contact with infected animals as domestic or production animal, and food consumption, which is the most important pathway. The clinical manifestation of the disease can have from mild to severe symptoms, including watery diarrhea (sometimes with blood), abdominal pain, fever, headache, nausea and to progressive paralysis that can result in respiratory failure and severe neurological dysfunction and may even lead to death. The occurrence of campylobacteriosis outbreaks requires immediate notification to the surveillance authorities, in order to initiate the investigation of common sources and transmission control through preventive measures, thereby minimizing the potential risks to human health.

Chapter 5 – *mpylobacter coli*, is among the main causes of bacterial gastroenteritis worldwide. In developing countries, campylobacteriosis is primarily a disease that occurs during infancy, because of high levels of early exposure and acquired immunity, but in industrialized countries, the epidemiology is characterized by sporadic infection throughout the population at all ages. The consumption of undercooked poultry, unpasteurized milk, improperly treated surface water and traveling abroad are the main sources of human campylobacter infection. Most infections are self-limiting, but antibiotic treatment may be required in cases of prolonged or severe illness and for vulnerable individuals, such as the very young or the very old. An increase in rates of resistance to fluoroquinolones in campylobacter stains from humans has been found associated with the approval of the use of fluoroquinolones (enrofloxacin) in veterinary medicine. Although there is no systematic surveillance and notification of Campylobacter infections in Greece, by retrieving data from various sources from general hospitals, *Campylobacter jejuni* is either the first or the second most common bacterial enteric pathogen (the other one being *Salmonella* ssp.) in our country. The last two decades several epidemiological studies that took place have delineated the epidemiology of Campylobacter in Greece. Serotyping studies have revealed that serotype HS:2 is the most predominant,whereas serotype HS:19 which is link to Guillain-Barré Syndrome (GBS), has also detected. Because of typing systems for Campylobacter epidemiologic studies vary in complexity and abilities to discriminate among strains versatile molecular surveys of characterization of Campylobacter strains based on *flaA* typing through RFLP led to the characterization of 39 differrent *flaA* types (*flaA*1-39 GR), whereas based on PFGE typing, a total of 43 different PFGE types were identified. MLST typing in conjunction with phylogenetic analysis revealed a total of 41 different MLST- sequence types of which 12 were unique in Greece. The studies also demonstrated that *racR* was the gene with the highest prevalence in our strain database. Besides, the resistance to fluoroquinolones in greek strains was not connected with the transferable gene *qnr*A. In conclusion, the Campylobacter infections in Greece, a) there are no notifications about small or large outbreaks, only sporadic cases have been hitherto reported, b) there is no clonality of the isolated strains on molecular level, c) commercially available foods seem not to be transmission sources and d) resistance rates to various antimicrobials agents vary, with those to fluoroquinolones remaining high. The burden of acute disease caused by campylobacter is important and underscores the need to develop effective surveillance systems in order to prevent human illness throughout each link in the food chain.

Chapter 6 – Poultry meat contaminated with *Campylobacter jejuni* and *Campylobacter coli* is a major cause of campylobacteriosis worldwide. These *Campylobacter* species are commensal organisms in the intestinal tract of live poultry and can cross contaminate carcasses during slaughter and processing. A range of chemical disinfectants are used to reduce or eliminate *Campylobacter* on poultry and in the processing environment. Organic acids, inorganic phosphates and chlorine-based disinfectants are commonly used for this purpose with varying efficiency depending on the approach taken. Temperature, pH and the concentration of the disinfectants are important parameters in determining their effectiveness and it is also essential that they do not change the organoleptic properties of the meat. Specific compounds used include lactic acid, citric acid, sodium hypochlorite, acidified sodium chlorite, benzalkonium chloride and trisodium phosphate and many of these are of potential human health concern. Novel, potentially less toxic and more environmentally friendly compounds are continually being sought to address this issue. The mode of action, effectiveness and applicability of established and novel disinfectants for the control of *Campylobacter* in poultry processing facilities are critically reviewed.

In: Campylobacter Infections
Editor: Brittany A. Bertucci

ISBN: 978-1-63463-858-6

Chapter 1

A Review of *Campylobacter jejuni* Pathogenesis: Main Virulence Factors and Their Use As Biomarkers

***Ramila C. Rodrigues*[1,2*], *Vicky Bronnec*[1,2*], *Odile Tresse*[1,2], *Jean-Michel Cappelier*[1,2] *and Nabila Haddad*[1,2†]**

[1]INRA UMR 1014 SECALIM, Nantes, France
[2]LUNAM Université, Oniris, Nantes, France

Abstract

Campylobacter jejuni is the leading cause of bacterial enteritis in the world and this zoonotic disease is mainly transmitted by food and water. *Campylobacter* infections are characterized by several symptoms such as watery/bloody diarrhea, abdominal pain, fever, headache, nausea and vomiting, which may persist for a few days. Post-infection complications

* These authors (R. C. Rodrigues and V. Bronnec) contributed equally to this work and should be considered co-first authors.

† Corresponding author: Nabila Haddad, UMR1014 SECALIM, Oniris, Route de Gachet, 44300 Nantes. Phone: 0033240684057; Fax: 0033251785520; email: nabila.haddad@oniris-nantes.fr.

are also observed, principally neurological disorders (Guillain-Barré syndrome) or reactive arthritis.

Many factors involved in *Campylobacter* virulence have been described in the literature. However, their intervention in the pathogenesis mechanism is still being investigated and their connections with the clinical signs of disease have not been clearly determined. Among the well-characterized virulence factors are flagella, responsible for motility and type III secretion of effectors, and intestinal colonization. In addition to the putative adhesins and invasins, the lipooligosaccharide (LOS) is involved in adhesion to/invasion of host cells and the mimicking of ganglioside sugars. The mechanisms of other virulence factors, such as the Cia proteins (*Campylobacter* invasion antigens) involved in invasion and the type VI secretion system recently described as interacting with the host, are not fully understood. Epidemiological analyses have revealed that the majority of genes encoding for virulence factors are present in the different *C. jejuni* strains, whatever their origin. Some of these genes contain inserted sequences or punctual mutations, which could be used as molecular tools to detect and identify *Campylobacter* spp.. Despite scientific advances concerning *C. jejuni* during the last decade, the knowledge and understanding of the virulence mechanisms of *Campylobacter* need further research. The objective here is to review the consensus virulence factors of *C. jejuni* pathogenesis in order to contribute to the risk management strategies for this foodborne pathogen and identify potential avenues to detect robust virulence factors.

Introduction

Campylobacters were first described in 1886 by Theodor Escherich, who observed spiral-shaped bacteria in stool samples of children suffering from diarrhea [1]. In the veterinary field, this bacterium has been known as a pathogen for more than a century [2]. In the early twentieth century, McFadyean and Stockman (1913) isolated bacteria close to the *Vibrio* genus from epizootic abortions in ewes while Smith (1919) isolated similar bacteria from bovine abortions [2, 3]. They called these bacteria *Vibrio fetus* [2, 3] mainly based on their screw-like shape. Then, diarrhea developed by cattle was attributed to *Vibrio*-like bacteria called *Vibrio jejuni*, while *Vibrio coli* was isolated from pigs harboring diarrhea [4, 5]. The first incidence of group *Campylobacter* poisoning in humans was observed in 1938 in a prison population in Illinois (USA). *Vibrio jejuni* were cultured from the blood of 13 sick prisoners and the milk distributed to prisoners [6]. Based on the GC percentage of the DNA sequence, Sebald and Veron distinguished the *Vibrio* genus from a new one: *Campylobacter* [7]. The analysis of *Campylobacter* since the 1970s has been facilitated by the development of cultivation techniques and selective media, which have enabled their identification in routine checks. Having been initially related to the *Vibrio* genus, it took almost a century between the first observation of this bacterium by Escherich and recognition of the importance of *Campylobacter* from a clinical, ecological and economic point of view [8, 9].

Campylobacter is a Gram-negative motile bacterium characterized by its obligate microaerobic feature. This genus belongs to the family of *Campylobacteraceae*, which also includes *Arcobacter* and *Sulfurospirillum* [10]. The genus *Campylobacter* is comprised of several species isolated from human and animal cases. However, to date, those most commonly isolated from foodborne disease are the thermophilic species *C. jejuni* and *C. coli* [11]. The exact contribution of these two species to the human disease burden varies with the setting and over time, but approximately 90% of cases are caused by *C. jejuni* and 10% by *C. coli* [11]. These organisms are widespread in the gut of farmed and wild animals and can be isolated from various environmental reservoirs, principally the digestive tract of wild and domesticated birds and mammals. These bacteria are prevalent in food-producing animals such as poultry, cattle, pigs and sheep and, to a lesser extent, in pets, wild birds and environmental water sources [11]. Animals rarely succumb to the disease caused by these organisms [11]. The human enteritis caused by *Campylobacter* sp. is called campylobacteriosis. According to the EFSA report (2014), *Campylobacter* has been the most commonly reported zoonotic agent in humans in the EU since 2005 [11]. Patients may experience mild to severe symptoms, with common clinical symptoms including watery, sometimes bloody diarrhea, abdominal pain, fever, headache and nausea. Infections are usually self-limiting and last only a few days. Post-infection complications, such as reactive arthritis and neurological disorders, can also occur. Nowadays, *C. jejuni* has become the most commonly recognized antecedent cause of Guillain–Barré syndrome, a polio-like form of paralysis that can result in respiratory failure and severe neurological dysfunction and even death [11].

In contrast to chicken gut colonization, *C. jejuni* in the human digestive tract have to achieve both colonization and internalization to cause infection. For an efficient infection, this pathogen must fulfill several conditions, including high motility [12] to overcome the detrimental effects of bile, the expression of adhesion molecules [13, 14] and survival of the antimicrobial effect of human serum in the case of a systemic infection [15]. The mechanisms by which *Campylobacter* species cause diarrhea, and possible sequelae, are not well defined. Four important pathogenic stages have been identified: (i) colonization of the digestive tract, (ii) adhesion to and invasion of intestinal cells, (iii) production of toxins.

Many factors involved in virulence have been described in the literature. For some, their role in colonization, adhesion to or invasion of host cells is well documented. However, for most, their intervention in the pathogenesis mechanism of *Campylobacter* has not been fully demonstrated and their relationships with the clinical signs of disease have not been clearly determined. The objective of the current review is to discuss the involvement of the main virulence factors in the pathogenic mechanism of *C. jejuni* and their use as biomarkers to detect and identify the pathogen.

Colonization of the Digestive Tract and Adhesion of *C. jejuni* to Human Epithelial Cells

As a zoonotic pathogen, *Campylobacter* colonizes the gastrointestinal tracts of a variety of animal hosts, either as a commensal or as a pathogen. Understanding the colonization mechanisms of *Campylobacter* is necessary to set up control strategies.

1. Motility: Chemotaxis and Flagellar Apparatus

C. jejuni is a highly motile pathogen and chemotaxis is an important factor in its pathogenesis. Chemotaxis is defined as the ability to detect and to move according to a chemical gradient: attraction to nutrients and repulsion by toxins. This specific motion of C. *jejuni* favors its survival and its colonization of the intestinal mucosa. A non-chemotactic mutant is unable to colonize the gastrointestinal tract of animals [16]. Several components of the C. *jejuni* chemotaxis system have been identified, including the genes *che*A, *che*B, *che*R, *che*Y, *che*V and *che*W and 10 other chemoreceptors [17]. The methylesterase CheB and methyltransferase CheR are both involved in chemotaxis as demonstrated by using a double mutant Δ*che*BR, whose ability to colonize the chicken cecum was reduced [18, 19]. CheY appears important for activating the rotation of the flagellum [19]. In addition to its role in the invasion process and general modulation of the virulence gene in *C. jejuni* [20, 21], a mutant with a deleted cheY gene showed a decrease in its ability to colonize chicken ceca [22].

Flagellar motility is one factor of *C. jejuni* required for both commensal colonization of poultry and infection of humans [12, 22-25]. Moreover, flagella are essential for the survival of *C. jejuni* under different environmental conditions [24], particularly when the pathogen is found in the digestive tract where the viscosity of the medium promotes bacterial motility [26]. *C. jejuni* moves by a spiral motion (corkscrew) via one or two unsheathed polar flagella, which participate in entering and colonizing the intestinal mucosa [27, 28]. The importance of the flagella in colonization and/or infection has been demonstrated in many organisms and also among different species of *Campylobacter* [29]. The inactivation of the *fla*A gene in C. *jejuni* leads to a reduction in bacterial motility [26] and a deficiency in its capacity to colonize the digestive tract of chickens [30].

Regulation of the *C. jejuni* virulence gene is not well documented; however, several two-component regulatory systems (TCRS) have been identified in *C. jejuni* as important for optimal chick colonization. The RacRS signal transduction system was the first described in *C. jejuni* [31]. This system responds to temperature variations and a mutation of the *rac*R gene reduced the potential of *C. jejuni* to colonize 1-day-old chicks [31]. Besides its role in the optimal colonization of chick gut, *C. jejuni* DccRS was found to be important for colonization by eliciting inflammation in the SCID-LF limited flora mouse model [32, 33]. Thus the SCID-LF inflammation analyses suggest a role for *dcc*RS in disease aetiology as well [32]. Among them, CprRS could control essential biological processes, stress tolerance and biofilm formation, resulting in a potential fitness of *C. jejuni* to adapt to various environments [34]. A Δ*cpr*S mutant was reported to display a dramatic dose-dependent defect for chick colonization [34]. Although these systems are not specific for host digestive tract colonization by *C. jejuni*, it is clear that this pathogen harbors multiple TCRS genes, involved in all aspects of its biology, which are vital for its efficient adaptation to the host.

2. Main Putative Adhesion Factors

Adhesion to epithelial cells is an essential step in bacterial infection. It is a prerequisite to colonize the host intestine and invade epithelial cells. This step usually involves surface structures such as pili or fimbriae; however, some studies have reported the absence of such structures in *C. jejuni* [17, 35]. As a result, several putative adhesion factors have been characterized and their role in adhesion to intestinal cells highlighted.

The most studied protein is CadF (*Campylobacter* adhesion to fibronectin), which is a glycoprotein of the extracellular matrix that binds to membrane-spanning receptor proteins called integrins. Inactivation of the *cad*F gene in *C. jejuni* leads to a 50% reduction in adhesion to human cells INT-407 of the mutant strain and a fall in chicken gut colonization [36, 37]. Moreover, this virulence factor contributes to the complex process of *C. jejuni* adhesion to inert surfaces, which is a preliminary step for biofilm formation, as revealed by a reduction in the capability of *C. jejuni* 81–176 Δ*cad*F cells compared to the isogenic strain [38].

In addition to CadF, FlpA (*cj1279c*) and the protein encoded by *cj1349c* have also been reported to contain fibronectin-type III domains and to act as fibronectin and fibrinogen-binding proteins, suggesting a close interaction with eukaryotic cells [13]. *C. jejuni* can bind to host cells via another adhesin called PEB1, which belongs to the cell-binding factor family. Deletion of the *peb*1 gene induces a 50- to 100-fold decrease in *C. jejuni* adhesion to epithelial cells [39]. Moreover, the mutant strain has a reduced colonization rate and duration in mice [39]. Recent studies demonstrate that PEB1 does not appear to act as an adhesin but rather has a critical role in aspartate and glutamate transport. Considering that amino acids are the unique carbon source of this asaccharolytic bacterium, amino acid transport is essential for *C. jejuni* colonization *in vivo* and persistence in the chicken gut [13]. Other proteins of the PEB family have been described in *C. jejuni*. For instance, Peb4 was shown to be involved in the adhesion of *C. jejuni* to eukaryotic cells through exporting proteins, such as CadF, into the outer membrane, [40-42].

However, inactivation of *cad*F and *peb*1 genes does not completely abolish adhesion of *C. jejuni* to the host cells, suggesting that other structures are also involved in this phenomenon. Ashgar et al. (2007) identified a putative autotransporter, which was termed CapA (*Campylobacter* adhesion protein A). *C. jejuni cap*A is a contingency gene, in which expression of the functional protein is dependent upon frameshifts within a homopolymeric nucleotide tract located near the 5'-end of the *cap*A coding region [43]. A *C. jejuni cap*A mutant demonstrated a reduction in adherence to human Caco-2 colorectal adenocarcinoma epithelial cells and a decrease in the efficient colonization of chickens [43].

The lipoprotein JlpA is also involved in adhesion of *C. jejuni* to Hep-2 cells. This protein interacts with HSP90, which is located at the surface of eukaryotic cells, and activates the NF-κβ pathway and the p38 MAP kinase resulting in a proinflammatory response [44, 45]. However, an insertional mutagenesis in *jlp*A gene did not result in a reduction in binding to chicken LMH cells [13]. In agreement with the results from the in vitro binding assays, the *jlp*A mutant was able to colonize broiler chickens at a comparable level to that of a parental isolate [13].

As colonization is a multifactorial process dependent on motility, chemotaxis, and the synthesis of multiple adhesins, Flanagan et al. (2009) evaluated the contribution of adhesins, including CadF and PEB1, in *C. jejuni*-host cell interactions *in vivo* [13]. They found that the *C. jejuni* CadF, CapA, FlpA, and Cj1349c proteins contributed to the bacterium in vitro adherence to chicken LMH, hepatocellular carcinoma epithelial cells, while CadF, PEB1, and FlpA contributed to the bacterium *in vivo* colonization of broiler chicks [13]. Moreover, commensal colonization of chicks seems to require expression of the invasin CiaI and Feds proteins, which is dependent on the σ^{28} factor [46].

3. Effect of the Mucus on *C. jejuni* Gut Colonization

The physical organization and composition of the mucus layer (mostly constituted of glycoproteins, intestinal microbiota and antimicrobial peptides) protect the epithelial cells from pathogenic bacteria. Thus, to cause disease, enteric pathogens have to colonize and destroy the mucus. Typically, they break down the mucus layer by secreting mucus degradative enzymes, such as mucinases, sialidases, N-acetyl-neuraminatelyases, glycosulfatases and sialate o-acetylesterases. In addition, chemotaxis and flagellar motility facilitate colonization and penetration of the mucus barrier by enteric pathogens, especially *C. jejuni*. Moreover, highly viscous solutions facilitate the motility of *C. jejuni* and this is correlated with an increased virulence potential of the pathogen *in vitro*. Pre-incubation of *C. jejuni* in media of higher viscosity enhanced bacterial binding and internalization into Caco-2 human cells [28].

The spiral shape of *C. jejuni* and the relatively short O-side chains of its lipooligosaccharides (LOS) are thought to prevent non-specific binding of this pathogen to mucin glycoproteins [47]. In addition, it was demonstrated that *C. jejuni* is able to grow in chicken and human mucus [48, 49]. Moreover, using a mucin microarray containing a wide range of natural mucins, including those from a number of gastrointestinal locations in different animal species, Naughton et al. (2013) demonstrated that *C. jejuni* showed a marked tropism for mucin obtained from chicken intestine [50]. These data suggest an adaptation of these bacteria to the mucus environment, conferring on *C. jejuni* an ecological advantage to outcompete native flora *in vivo*.

Beside the fact that *C. jejuni* must break the protective mucus layer, it appears that this barrier could even enhance bacterial pathogenicity. Alemka et al. (2010) showed that, compared with parental HT29 human cells without mucus secretion, bacterial binding and internalization were promoted by E12-producing mucus cells [50, 51]. Moreover, Tu et al. (2008) revealed that the presence of MUC2 (the main intestinal gel-forming mucin) upregulated some *C. jejuni* virulence genes, including those involved in motility (*fla*A), adhesion (*jlp*A), invasion (*cia*B), and toxin formation (*cdt*) [52]. In contrast, *C. jejuni* in contact with purified chicken mucus led to a decrease in virulence of the bacteria [48]. Similarly, crude chicken intestinal mucus attenuated *C. jejuni* binding and internalization into chicken epithelial cells [53]. These contradictory results could be explained by the mucus composition, and especially the presence of sulfated mucin glycoproteins, which can affect *C. jejuni* mucus colonization and pathogenicity. These data indicate that mucus and mucins modulate *C. jejuni* virulence and may contribute to the different clinical manifestations exhibited by this pathogen in different hosts.

4. Resistance to Antibiotics and Fitness *In Vivo*

Colonization of the host gastrointestinal tract is closely linked to the ability of the pathogen to survive antimicrobial substances *in vivo*. As a zoonotic pathogen, *C. jejuni* is highly prevalent in food products from farm animals, mainly poultry, and is subjected to animal antibiotherapies. Although there is controlled use of antibiotics in poultry production, fluoroquinolone-resistant *Campylobacter* resist several rotations on poultry farms suggesting that these strains do not show a fitness cost in the absence of antibiotic selection pressure and are ecologically competitive in farm environments [54-56]. In *C. jejuni*, resistance to fluoroquinolone is mediated by point mutations in the DNA gyrase-encoding gene *gyr*A [57]. Resistance-conferring mutations in target genes are often associated with changes in physiological processes, which may result in reduced growth and fitness in the absence of antibiotics [58]. However, *C. jejuni*, like many other bacteria, has developed compensatory mutations to improve the fitness cost associated with antimicrobial resistance. In fact, when co-inoculated into chickens, the fluoroquinolone-resistant *Campylobacter* isolates outcompete the fluoroquinolone-susceptible strains, indicating that acquisition of fluoroquinolone-resistance enhances the *in vivo* fitness of *Campylobacter* [59, 60]. In contrast to fluoroquinolone, the acquisition of macrolide resistance impairs the fitness and transmission of *Campylobacter* in chickens, suggesting that the prevalence of macrolide-resistant *C. jejuni* will probably decrease in the absence of antibiotic selection pressure [61, 62].

The current survival of fluoroquinolone-resistant *Campylobacter* threatens clinical treatments and could affect the health of human hosts. Several studies reported that human patients infected by fluoroquinolone-resistant *Campylobacter* had prolonged diarrhea, increased risk of invasive illness and hospitalization compared with patients infected with fluoroquinolone-susceptible strains [63, 64]. However, no study has indicated if this increased clinical severity is the consequence of the enhanced virulence of these mutant strains or a treatment failure.

Invasion of Human Intestinal Cells by *C. jejuni* and Crossing the Epithelial Barrier

During infection of humans, epithelial cell invasion is a major determinant of *C. jejuni* virulence. *C. jejuni* invasion of intestinal and colonic epithelial cells is thought to contribute to inflammation and destruction of the epithelium [65]. Both invasion and the host inflammatory response participate in pathogenesis. Moreover, invasion studies using intestinal epithelial cells revealed a statistically significant correlation between the ability of *C. jejuni* to invade cultured cells and the severity of the clinical symptoms of infection [66].

1. Flagella and Secreted Proteins

Human host cell invasion by *C. jejuni* may involve additive effects of proteins involved in cell adhesion. For example, CadF and FlpA adhesins may act together to target fibronectin for bacterial binding and subsequent invasion by *C. jejuni* [67]. However, studies have revealed that de novo bacterial protein synthesis is required for maximal *C. jejuni* invasion [68, 69]. Therefore, constitutive expression of these adhesins alone is not sufficient for the bacterial uptake process [67, 70].

Among proteins synthesized *de novo* and involved in the invasion mechanism, Cia (*Campylobacter* invasin antigen) proteins play a major role. Flagella and flagellar motility are required for invasion of human intestinal epithelial cells [21, 71, 72]. In addition to protein secretion for flagellar biosynthesis, the *C. jejuni* flagellar type III secretion system (T3SS) is involved in the secretion of proteins required for interactions with eukaryotic cells, including Cia proteins [73-76]. Moreover, Neal McKinney and Konkel (2012) demonstrated that the delivery of *C. jejuni* Cia proteins into human INT407 epithelial cells required a functional flagellar hook complex composed of FlgE, FlgK, and FlgL [77]. Synthesis of Cia proteins has been reported to be induced by bile salts, with flagellum-dependent secretion of these proteins requiring either a factor produced by intestinal cells or components of serum [74, 78, 79]. In addition, CiaC is released into host cells by cell-associated (bound) bacteria [77]. *C. jejuni* mutant strains lacking Cia proteins (CiaB, CiaC, CiaD and CiaI) have less ability to invade or survive within eukaryotic cells [70, 73, 80, 81]. More precisely, a recent work indicated that CiaI is not required for *C. jejuni* internalization into host cells, but seems essential for the pathogen to facilitate commensal colonization of the chicken digestive tract [82].

Other proteins of *C. jejuni*, such as FlaC and FspA proteins, are secreted by the flagellum but are not dependent on bile salts for their expression or serum for their secretion. Interestingly, FlaC, a flagellin-like protein involved in motility, is required for full invasion of eukaryotic cells [76]. Two related FspA proteins are produced by different *C. jejuni* strains and FspA2 seems to promote apoptosis of eukaryotic cells [75].

2. *Campylobacter* Cia Proteins and Clinical Signs in Hosts

Of at least 18 Cia proteins detected in *C. jejuni*, only four (CiaB, CiaC, CiaD and CiaI) have been characterized to date [70, 77, 80, 81, 83]. While the precise functions of these proteins are not fully known, *in vivo* studies suggest that they are associated with the clinical signs of campylobacteriosis. For instance, the inoculation of piglets with a *C. jejuni cia*B mutant resulted in different clinical signs [83, 84]. Piglets infected with *C. jejuni* developed diarrhea within 24 h and exhibited severe histological lesions, whereas piglets inoculated with a *C. jejuni cia*B-knockout mutant strain did not develop diarrhea until 3 days post-infection and exhibited only minor histological lesions [83].

Furthermore, Samuelson et al. (2013) showed that CiaD is required for the development of acute disease *in vivo* in IL-10 knockout mice [81]. The *C. jejuni* wild-type strain resulted in disease characterized by a thickening of the gastrointestinal tract wall, enlarged ileocecocolic lymph nodes, and bloody lumen contents in the cecum and colon, which was absent in mice infected with the *C. jejuni cia*D mutant [81]. Further analyses are needed to identify and characterize the Cia proteins to gain a better understanding of *C. jejuni* pathogenesis.

3. Invasion Mechanism

Eucker and Konkel (2012) described a model in which an invasion complex enables the maximal internalization of host cells by *C. jejuni* [67]. This complex seems to involve *C. jejuni* CadF and FlpA adhesins and the T3SS-flagella secreting Cia proteins. Host cell proteins are also involved in this complex, such as FAK, paxillin, c-Src, Dock180 and Rac1, which appear to be key components [67, 85]. A model of the signal pathway leading to *C. jejuni* invasion was proposed by Eucker and Konkel (2012) [67]. Briefly, CadF and FlpA adhesins on the surface of *C. jejuni* bind to fibronectin and result in the activation of $\alpha5\beta1$ integrin receptors [85]. This interaction triggers FAK, which, associated with c-Src, induces paxillin and p130Cas activation [67, 85]. The adaptor protein p130Cas recruits Dock180, which participates in the activation of Rac1, the Rho family monomeric G protein [67, 85]. *C. jejuni* Cia proteins are also responsible for Rho GTPase Rac1 recruitment and activation, resulting in a local restructuring of the cytoskeleton [67, 77, 85, 86]. Activation of the *C. jejuni* invasion complex ultimately leads to *C. jejuni* uptake, where membrane ruffling is triggered in response to Rac1 activation. In addition to this model, Bouwan et al. (2013) revealed a novel internalization process in polarized epithelial cells via an actin- and microtubule-independent process [87]. However, it is not yet clear which mechanism of internalization, "zipper" or "trigger", is used by *C. jejuni*. As mentioned above, several studies have indicated that *C. jejuni* induces membrane ruffling in a contact-dependent manner (via CadF and FlpA adhesins), followed by introduction of the flagella-T3SS into the host cell cytoplasm delivering Cia proteins. This interaction leads to recruitment and activation of the *C. jejuni* invasion complex [67, 88]. All together, these steps promote an activation of the host cell signaling pathway leading to cytoskeleton remodeling and pathogen entry. Surprisingly, these different results indicate that the *C. jejuni* invasion mechanism shares some features of both the “zipper” and “trigger” mechanisms.

Once inside host cells, *C. jejuni* is able to cross polarized intestinal epithelial cells, entering deeper tissues and causing short- or long-term infections in the human body. This phenomenon may involve either paracellular or transcellular routes. In the case of *C. jejuni*, the literature is highly controversial. While some groups report the paracellular route, others describe the transcellular model or a mix of both [71, 89-93]. More recently, Boehm et al. (2012) argued for the paracellular route and demonstrated the role of HtrA protease in the transmigration of *C. jejuni* across polarized epithelial cells without affecting the transepithelial electrical resistance [94].

4. Other Surface Structures Involved in *C. jejuni* Internalization in Host Cells

Structures such as lipooligosaccharides (LOS) confer variable virulence-associated phenotypes on *C. jejuni*. Inactivation of *gal*E (encoding a UDP-glucose 4-epimerase) or *waa*F (encoding heptosyltransferase II) results in microorganisms expressing deeply truncated LOS molecules and with a reduced potential to invade epithelial cells *in vitro* [95]. Furthermore, complete deletion of the LOS biosynthesis locus in *C. jejuni* NCTC11168 decreased growth and induced the loss of invasion and natural transformation efficiency of the mutant [96]. In addition, the sialylated lipooligosaccharide of the *Campylobacter* cell wall is associated with an increased occurrence of bloody diarrhea and the late onset complication of Guillain-Barré syndrome [96-99].

However, there are conflicting reports about the universal requirement of LOS proteins for cell invasion among different *C. jejuni* strains. Strains with mutations in *cgt*A, which encodes an outer core N-acetylgalactosaminyltransferase in *C. jejuni* 81-176, exhibited increased bacterial attachment and invasion of human cells while, in the same study, mutation of *neu*C1, leading to the absence of sialic acid in the outer core, had no effect on invasiveness [100]. These studies indicate that a minimal LOS core structure is required for optimal invasion and mutations occurring in this sequence impair invasion [101]. Mutations outside the core (e.g., *cgt*A) are more likely to have strain-specific effects on invasion.

In addition, a type VI secretion system (T6SS) was described in *C. jejuni*. Lertpiriyapong et al. (2012) demonstrated that the human clinical isolate *C. jejuni* ATCC43431 contains a T6SS gene cluster that encodes a functional secretion system. In vitro analyses revealed that T6SS isogenic mutants displayed an approximately 50% reduction in cell adhesion and invasion compared to the parental strain [102]. Their results were complemented by *in vivo* studies demonstrating the importance of T6SS in establishing persistent colonization [102]. Moreover, it was shown that T6SS is present in about 10% of *C. jejuni* strains, including several blood isolates [103].

Cytotoxicity of *C. jejuni*

Supposed *C. jejuni* toxins include (i) a cytolethal distending toxin (CDT), (ii) a cholera toxin-like enterotoxin (CTLT), (iii) and a number of cytotoxins [104]. However, only the genes encoding the CDT have been identified and characterized. There is uncertainty about the production of CTLT by C. jejuni [105], while Gatsos et al. (2012) have attempted to characterize the unknown cytotoxins [106]. After an activity assay based on the lethal effects of the toxin on CHO cells to screen rapidly for activity, these authors purified the bacterial supernatant by chromatographic analyses to identify active proteins [106]. Unexpectedly, they found some previously uncharacterized non-cytoplasmic proteins, which might be attributable to cytotoxins. The activity of the toxin-containing fraction was validated by performing the rabbit ileal loop assay. Further analyses are required to confirm the role of these new *C. jejuni* cytotoxins [106].

Concerning the CDT, the genes encoding this toxin (*cdt*A/B/C) have been detected and CDT is the best characterized toxin in *C. jejuni*. It is also produced by *Escherichia coli*, *Shigella* spp., and *Helicobacter hepaticus*, and is responsible for cell cycle arrest in the G_2 phase by degrading DNA, causing progressive cellular distension with eventual cell death [107-110]. Three subunits compose the functional CDT holotoxin. CdtA and CdtC interact with the eukaryotic cell membrane promoting the internalization of the subunit CdtB. Then, CdtB, which contains a DNase activity, cleaves the chromosome, resulting in the divided cell cycle arrest [111].

The DNA damage induced by *C. jejuni* CDT seems to have various effects according to the host cell line [112]. In epithelial cells, production of CDT by *C. jejuni* induces the production of interleukin IL-8, which activates the NF-kB pathway and the recruitment of dendritic cells, macrophages and neutrophils in the infection site [112, 113]. This interaction with *C. jejuni* may initiate inflammation of the intestine and diarrheal symptoms, at least in a mouse model [114]. Although the release of proinflammatory chemokines from infected monocytes appears to be independent of CDT, the cytotoxic effect is manifested by apoptosis [112].

C. jejuni CDT should not be neglected as a virulence attribute. Biswas et al. (2006) have shown that CDT does not play a role in the adhesion to both human and avian cells or in poultry gut colonization [115]. However, this toxin was shown to be involved in the internalization and/or survival of the pathogen in host cells [115]. This was confirmed by Jain et al. (2007) who showed that CDT-positive *C. jejuni* strains invade epithelial cells more efficiently than strains lacking *cdt*B genes [114].

Molecular Epidemiology and Virulence Genetic Markers

The identification of virulence genetic markers enables the development of molecular methods based on these genes and provides new tools for enhanced surveillance and outbreak detection. Several alternative and rapid methods have been developed to detect and confirm *Campylobacter* spp. To date, the most effective confirmation methods are based on uncultured assays using the PCR reaction.

Although various studies have shown that the *cad*F gene is detected using PCR in *C. jejuni* and *C. coli* isolates from different countries [116-121], Krause-Gruszczynska et al. (2007) observed that all *C. coli* isolates tested possessed a larger CadF than *C. jejuni*, with an additional stretch of 7 to 13 amino acids in the protein. This difference between the *C. jejuni* and *C. coli* isolates could be a suitable diagnostic marker to discriminate these species in food and clinical specimens [122].

The *cad*F gene is not the only virulence biomarker suggested to track *C. jejuni*. In order to determine the distribution of some genetic markers and their correlation with the clinical data observed, Zautner et al. (2012) characterized 266 isolates [123]. They described two major types of marker gene combinations represented by group 1A and group 2B. All other groups depicted a gradual transition of marker gene combinations between these two groups. Group 1A is better adapted to livestock and characterized by the ability to use L-fucose and the presence of all of the five identified putative *C. jejuni* iron-uptake systems as well as the flagellin O-glycosylation locus (*cj1321-cj1326*), *cj1365c*, *cj1585c*, and sialylated LOS genes (*cst*II and/or *cst*III) [123]. These isolates do not exhibit the genes for an extended amino acid metabolism. Due to their livestock adaptation, they are less prevalent in humans and secondarily associated with less severe campylobacterioses [123]. In contrast, group 2B isolates possess an extended amino acid metabolism (positive for *ans*B, *dms*A, and *ggt*) and are unable to metabolize L-fucose (*fuc*P-negative). They are related to a higher prevalence in human campylobacteriosis, bloody diarrhea and hospitalization and clearly have a higher virulence for humans [123].

Several epidemiological studies have also focused on the detection of *cdt* genes in *C. jejuni* isolates from animals. They revealed the high prevalence of these genes in both *C. jejuni* and *C. coli* isolates from poultry and food samples [119, 124, 125]. However, the percentage of homology of each *cdt* gene varies between *C. jejuni*, *C. coli* and *C. fetus* species from 70% for the *cdt*B gene between *C. jejuni* and *C. coli* to 40% for *cdt*A between *C. jejuni* and *C. fetus* [126]. This comparison enables species-specific primers to be defined in order to develop molecular methods for the routine identification of *Campylobacter* species in clinical laboratories. For example, *cdt* genes have been targeted to develop a species-specific multiplex PCR for the detection and identification of *Campylobacter* spp. from different samples, such as stool specimens of patients with gastroenteritis symptoms or food [127-130]. The results highlight the rapidity and sensitivity of this molecular method in comparison with the culture method usually used [130].

Moreover, virulence genes are used for epidemiological typing methods leading to the characterization and discrimination of bacterial strains. The data are used for public health surveillance, disease cluster identification and outbreak investigations. Because of its significant sequence heterogeneity, the flagellin-encoding *fla*A gene has been used in the epidemiological typing of *Campylobacter* isolates as the target for PCR-RFLP typing, and sequencing of a short variable region [131-133]. The *fla*A gene is recommended as a good epidemiological marker for molecular analysis and the *fla*A-RFLP is one of the simplest and most cost-effective methods for the investigation of large numbers of isolates.

Conclusion

In contrast to other invasive foodborne bacterial pathogens, including *Listeria monocytogenes* [134], *Salmonella enterica* [135] and *Staphylococcus aureus* [136], the molecular mechanisms of *C. jejuni* invasion remain elusive. In *C. jejuni*, some factors have been demonstrated to contribute to sporadic illnesses. However, a defined biochemical pathway of translocation or internalization into host cells has not yet been discovered. *C. jejuni* virulence still puzzles scientists, as the underlying molecular mechanisms seem to be unique to this pathogen, without sharing any common factors that have been identified in other foodborne pathogens except fibronectin-binding proteins. Although recent advances concerning *S. enterica* and *S. aureus* have described novel host cell invasion strategies [137, 138] or new signaling effectors of the infectious process of *L. monocytogenes* [139], the elucidation of *Campylobacter* infection is still at an early stage. Nevertheless, some significant illness promoters described as virulence factors in *Campylobacter* could be used solely or in combination as biological markers to pinpoint the virulence at the level of the species or the strain. As bacterial physiopathology is human cell feature-dependent, the limited number of animal models available for *Campylobacter* infection represents the most difficult issue to be addressed. The challenges for future studies include (i) a better understanding of the routes of *C. jejuni* infection and (ii) the determination of consensus molecular phenomena of invasion among the multigenetic variability of strains.

References

[1] Escherich, T., Beitrage zur Kenntniss der Darmbactrien. III. Ueber das Vorkommen von Vibrionen im Darmcanal und den Stuhlgangen der Sauglinge. *Münchener Medizinische Wochenschrift*, 1886. 33: p. 815-817.

[2] McFadyean, J. and S. Stockman, Report of the Departmental Committee appointed by the Board of Agriculture and Fisheries to inquire into epizootic abortion of sheep, in HMSO. 1913: London.

[3] Smith, T. and M. Taylor, Some morphological and biological characters of the spirilla (*Vibrio fetus*) associated with disease of the fetal membranes in cattle. *Journal of Experimental Medicine*, 1919. 30: p. 299-231.

[4] Doyle, L., A vibrio associated with swine dysentery. *American Journal of Veterinary Research*, 1944. 5: p. 3-5.

[5] Jones, F. and M. Orcutt, *Vibrio* (*Vibrio jejuni*) associated with intestinal disorders of cows and calves. *Journal of Experimental Medicine*, 1931. 53: p. 853-864.

[6] Levy, A., A gastro-enteritis outbreak probably due to a bovine strain of *Vibrio*. *Journal of Infectious Diseases*, 1946. 18: p. 243-258.

[7] Sebald, M. and M. Veron, Teneur en base de l'ADN et classification des vibrions. *Annales de l'Institut Pasteur*, 1963. 105: p. 897-910.

[8] Skirrow, M.B., John McFadyean and the centenary of the first isolation of *Campylobacter* species. *Clinical Infectious Diseases*, 2006. 43(9): p. 1213-1217.

[9] Snelling, W.J., et al., Under the microscope - *Campylobacter jejuni*. *Letters in Applied Microbiology*, 2005. 41(4): p. 297-302.

[10] Vandamme, P., et al., Revision of *Campylobacter*, *Helicobacter*, and *Wolinella* taxonomy: emendation of generic descriptions and proposal of *Arcobacter* gen. nov. *International Journal of Systematic Bacteriology*, 1991. 41(1): p. 88-103.

[11] Anonymous, The European Union summary report on trends and sources of zoonoses, zoonotic agents and food-borne outbreaks in 2012. *EFSA Journal,* 2014. 12(2): p. 3547, 312.

[12] Wassenaar, T.M., et al., Colonization of chicks by motility mutants of *Campylobacter jejuni* demonstrates the importance of flagellin-A expression. *Journal of General Microbiology*, 1993. 139: p. 1171-1175.

[13] Flanagan, R.C., et al., Examination of *Campylobacter jejuni* putative adhesins leads to the identification of a new protein, designated FlpA, required for chicken colonization. *Infection and Immunity*, 2009. 77(6): p. 2399-2407.

[14] Konkel, M.E., et al., *Campylobacter jejuni* strains compete for colonization in broiler chicks. *Applied and Environmental Microbiology*, 2007. 73: p. 2297-2305.

[15] Guerry, P., et al., Sialylation of lipooligosaccharide cores affects immunogenicity and serum resistance of *Campylobacter jejuni*. *Infection and Immunity*, 2000. 68(12): p. 6656-6662.

[16] Takata, T., S. Fujimoto, and K. Amako, Isolation of nonchemotactic mutants of *Campylobacter jejuni* and their colonization of the mouse intestinal tract. *Infection and Immunity*, 1992. 60(9): p. 3596-600.

[17] Parkhill, J., et al., The genome sequence of the food-borne pathogen *Campylobacter jejuni* reveals hypervariable sequences. *Nature*, 2000. 403(6770): p. 665-668.

[18] Kanungpean, D., T. Kakuda, and S. Takai, Participation of CheR and CheB in the chemosensory response of *Campylobacter jejuni*. *Microbiology,* 2011. 157(Pt 5): p. 1279-89.

[19] Stephens, B.B., S.N. Loar, and G. Alexandre, Role of CheB and CheR in the complex chemotactic and aerotactic pathway of Azospirillum brasilense. *Journal of Bacteriology*, 2006. 188(13): p. 4759-68.

[20] van Vliet, A.H., et al., The iron-induced ferredoxin FdxA of *Campylobacter jejuni* is involved in aerotolerance. *FEMS Microbiology Letters*, 2001. 196(2): p. 189-93.

[21] Yao, R.J., et al., Isolation of motile and nonmotile insertional mutants of *Campylobacter jejuni* - the role of motility in adherence and invasion of eukaryotic cells. *Molecular Microbiology*, 1994. 14(5): p. 883-893.

[22] Hendrixson, D.R. and V.J. DiRita, Identification of *Campylobacter jejuni* genes involved in commensal colonization of the chick gastrointestinal tract. *Molecular Microbiology*, 2004. 52(2): p. 471-484.

[23] Black, R.E., et al., Experimental *Campylobacter jejuni* infection in humans. *Journal of Infectious Diseases*, 1988. 157: p. 472-479.

[24] Nachamkin, I., X.H. Yang, and N.J. Stern, Role of *Campylobacter jejuni* flagella as colonization factors for 3-day-old chicks - analysis with flagellar mutants. *Applied and Environmental Microbiology*, 1993. 59(5): p. 1269-1273.

[25] Wosten, M.M., J.A. Wagenaar, and J.P. van Putten, The FlgS/FlgR two-component signal transduction system regulates the *fla* regulon in *Campylobacter jejuni*. *Journal of Biological Chemistry*, 2004. 279(16): p. 16214-22.

[26] Guerry, P., *Campylobacter* flagella: not just for motility. *Trends in Microbiology,* 2007. 15(10): p. 456-61.

[27] Newell, D.G., et al., Changes in the carriage of *Campylobacter* strains by poultry carcasses during processing in abattoirs. *Applied and Environmental Microbiology*, 2001. 67(6): p. 2636-2640.

[28] Szymanski, C.M., et al., *Campylobacter jejuni* motility and invasion of Caco-2 cells. *Infection and Immunity*, 1995. 63: p. 4295-4300.

[29] Nachamkin, I. and X.H. Yang, Local immune responses to the *Campylobacter* flagellin in acute *Campylobacter* gastrointestinal infection. *Journal of Clinical Microbiology*, 1992. 30(2): p. 509-11.

[30] Fields, P.I. and D.L. Swerdlow, *Campylobacter jejuni*. *Clinics Laboratory Medicine*, 1999. 19(3): p. 489-504, v.

[31] Bras, A.M., et al., A novel *Campylobacter jejuni* two-component regulatory system important for temperature-dependent growth and colonization. *Journal of Bacteriology*, 1999. 181(10): p. 3298-3302.

[32] MacKichan, J.K., et al., The *Campylobacter jejuni dcc*RS two-component system is required for optimal in vivo colonization but is

dispensable for in vitro growth. *Molecular Microbiology*, 2004. 54(5): p. 1269-1286.

[33] Wosten, M.M., et al., Growth phase-dependent activation of the DccRS regulon of *Campylobacter jejuni*. *Journal of Bacteriology*, 2010. 192(11): p. 2729-36.

[34] Svensson, S.L., et al., The CprS sensor kinase of the zoonotic pathogen *Campylobacter jejuni* influences biofilm formation and is required for optimal chick colonization. *Molecular Microbiology*, 2009. 71(1): p. 253-272.

[35] Fouts, D.E., et al., Major structural differences and novel potential virulence mechanisms from the genomes of multiple *Campylobacter* species. *Plos Biology*, 2005. 3(1): p. 72-85.

[36] Monteville, M.R., J.E. Yoon, and K.E. Konkel, Maximal adherence and invasion of INT 407 cells by *Campylobacter jejuni* requires the CadF outer membrane protein and microfilament reorganization. *Microbiology-Sgm*, 2003. 149: p. 153-165.

[37] Ziprin, R.L., et al., The absence of cecal colonization of chicks by a mutant of *Campylobacter jejuni* not expressing bacterial fibronectin-binding protein. *Avian Diseases*, 1999. 43(3): p. 586-589.

[38] Sulaeman, S., et al., Enhanced adhesion of *Campylobacter jejuni* to abiotic surfaces is mediated by membrane proteins in oxygen-enriched conditions. *PLoS One*, 2012. 7(9): p. e46402.

[39] Pei, Z.H., et al., Mutation in the *peb*1A locus of *Campylobacter jejuni* reduces interactions with epithelial cells and intestinal colonization of mice. *Infection and Immunity*, 1998. 66(3): p. 938-943.

[40] Asakura, H., et al., Deletion of *peb*4 gene impairs cell adhesion and biofilm formation in *Campylobacter jejuni*. *FEMS Microbiology Letters*, 2007. 275(2): p. 278-285.

[41] Kale, A., et al., The virulence factor PEB4 (Cj0596) and the periplasmic protein Cj1289 are two structurally related SurA-like chaperones in the human pathogen *Campylobacter jejuni*. *Journal of Biological Chemistry*, 2011. 286(24): p. 21254-65.

[42] Kervella, M., et al., Isolation and characterization of 2 *Campylobacter* glycine-extracted proteins that bind to Hela-cell membranes. *Infection and Immunity*, 1993. 61(8): p. 3440-3448.

[43] Ashgar, S.S., et al., CapA, an autotransporter protein of *Campylobacter* jejuni, mediates association with human epithelial cells and colonization of the chicken gut. *Journal of Bacteriology*, 2007. 189(5): p. 1856-65.

[44] Jin, S.M., et al., JlpA, a novel surface-exposed lipoprotein specific to *Campylobacter jejuni*, mediates adherence to host epithelial cells. *Molecular Microbiology*, 2001. 39(5): p. 1225-1236.

[45] Jin, S.M., et al., JlpA of *Campylobacter jejuni* interacts with surface-exposed heat shock protein 90 alpha and triggers signalling pathways leading to the activation of NF-kappa B and p38 MAP kinase in epithelial cells. *Cellular Microbiology*, 2003. 5(3): p. 165-174.

[46] Barrero-Tobon, A.M. and D.R. Hendrixson, Identification and analysis of flagellar coexpressed determinants (Feds) of *Campylobacter jejuni* involved in colonization. *Molecular Microbiology*, 2012. 84(2): p. 352-69.

[47] McSweegan, E. and R.I. Walker, Identification and characterization of two *Campylobacter jejuni* adhesins for cellular and mucous substrates. . *Infection and Immunity*, 1986. 53: p. 141-148.

[48] Alemka, A., et al., Purified chicken intestinal mucin attenuates *Campylobacter jejuni* pathogenicity *in vitro. Journal of Medical Microbiology,* 2010. 59: p. 898-903.

[49] Van Deun, K., et al., Colonization strategy of *Campylobacter jejuni* results in persistent infection of the chicken gut. *Veterinary Microbiology*, 2008. 130: p. 285-297.

[50] Naughton, J.A., et al., Divergent mechanisms of interaction of *Helicobacter pylori* and *Campylobacter jejuni* with mucus and mucins. Infection *and Immunity*, 2013. 81(8): p. 2838-50.

[51] Alemka, A., et al., Probiotic colonization of the adherent mucus layer of HT29MTXE12 cells attenuates *Campylobacter jejuni* virulence properties. *Infection and Immunity*, 2010. 78: p. 2812-2822.

[52] Tu, Q.V., M.A. Mc Guckin, and G.L. Mendz, *Campylobacter jejuni* response to human mucin MUC2: modulation of colonization and pathogenicity determinants. *Journal of Medical Microbiology*, 2008. 57: p. 795-802.

[53] Byrne, C.M., M. Clyne, and B. Bourke, *Campylobacter jejuni* adhere to and invade chicken intestinal epithelial cells *in vitro*. *Microbiology-Sgm,* 2007. 153: p. 561-569.

[54] Luangtongkum, T., et al., Antibiotic resistance in *Campylobacter*: emergence, transmission and persistence. *Future Microbiology*, 2009. 4(2): p. 189-200.

[55] Peterson, M.C., *Campylobacter jejuni* enteritis associated with consumption of raw milk. *Journal of Environmental Health*, 2003. 65(9): p. 20-1, 24, 26.

[56] Price, L.B., et al., The persistence of fluoroquinolone-resistant *Campylobacter* in poultry production. *Environmental Health Perspective*, 2007. 115(7): p. 1035-1039.

[57] Luo, N., et al., *In vivo* selection of *Campylobacter* isolates with high levels of fluoroquinolone resistance associated with *gyr*A mutations and the function of the CmeABC efflux pump. *Antimicrobial Agents Chemotherapy,* 2003. 47(1): p. 390-4.

[58] Levin, B.R., V. Perrot, and N. Walker, Compensatory mutations, antibiotic resistance and the population genetics of adaptive evolution in bacteria. *Genetic*s, 2000. 154(3): p. 985-97.

[59] Han, J., et al., A fluoroquinolone resistance associated mutation in *gyr*A Affects DNA supercoiling in *Campylobacter jejuni. Frontiers in Cellular and Infection Microbiology*, 2012. 2: p. 21.

[60] Luo, N., et al., Enhanced *in vivo* fitness of fluoroquinolone-resistant *Campylobacter jejuni* in the absence of antibiotic selection pressure. *Proceedings of the National Academy of Sciences of the United States of America*, 2005. 102(3): p. 541-6.

[61] Luangtongkum, T., et al., Impaired fitness and transmission of macrolide-resistant *Campylobacter jejuni* in its natural host. *Antimicrobial Agents and Chemotherapy*, 2012. 56(3): p. 1300-8.

[62] Zeitouni, S., et al., Fitness of macrolide resistant *Campylobacter coli* and *Campylobacter jejuni. Microbial Drug Resistance,* 2012. 18(2): p. 101-8.

[63] Engberg, J., et al., Quinolone-resistant Campylobacter infections: risk factors and clinical consequences. *Emerging Infectious Diseases*, 2004. 10(6): p. 1056-63.

[64] Helms, M., et al., Adverse health events associated with antimicrobial drug resistance in *Campylobacter* species: a registry-based cohort study. *Journal of Infectious Diseases*, 2005. 191(7): p. 1050-5.

[65] van Spreeuwel, J.P., et al., *Campylobacter colitis*: histological immunohistochemical and ultrastructural findings. *Gut,* 1985. 26: p. 945-951.

[66] Everest, P.H., et al., Differentiated Caco-2 cells as a model for enteric invasion by *Campylobacter jejuni* and *Campylobacter coli. Journal of Medical Microbiology*, 1992. 37(5): p. 319-325.

[67] Eucker, T.P. and M.E. Konkel, The cooperative action of bacterial fibronectin-binding proteins and secreted proteins promote maximal *Campylobacter jejuni* invasion of host cells by stimulating membrane ruffling. *Cellular Microbiology*, 2012. 14(2): p. 226-38.

[68] Konkel, M.E. and W. Cieplak, Altered synthetic response of *Campylobacter jejuni* to cocultivation with human epithelial-cells is associated with enhanced internalization. *Infection and Immunity*, 1992. 60(11): p. 4945-4949.

[69] Oelschlaeger, T.A., P. Guerry, and D.J. Kopecko, Unusual microtubule-dependent endocytosis mechanisms triggered by *Campylobacter jejuni* and *Citrobacter freundii. Proceedings of the National Academy of Sciences of the United States of America*, 1993. 90(14): p. 6884-6888.

[70] Christensen, J.E., S.A. Pacheco, and M.E. Konkel, Identification of a *Campylobacter jejuni*-secreted protein required for maximal invasion of host cells. *Molecular Microbiology*, 2009. 73(4): p. 650-662.

[71] Grant, C.C.R., et al., Role of flagella in adherence, internalisation, and translocation of *Campylobacter jejuni* in nonpolarized and polarized epithelial-cell cultures. *Infection and Immunity*, 1993. 61(5): p. 1764-1771.

[72] Wassenaar, T.M., N.M.C. Bleumink-Pluym, and B.A.M. Van der Zeijst, Inactivation of *Campylobacter jejuni* flagellin genes by homologous recombination demonstrates that *fla*A but not *fla*B is required for invasion. *The EMBO Journal*, 1991. 10(8): p. 2055-2061.

[73] Konkel, M.E., et al., Bacterial secreted proteins are required for the internalization of *Campylobacter jejuni* into cultured mammalian cells. *Molecular Microbiology*, 1999. 32(4): p. 691-701.

[74] Konkel, M.E., et al., Secretion of virulence proteins from *Campylobacter jejuni* is dependent on a functional flagellar export apparatus. *Journal of Bacteriology*, 2004. 186(11): p. 3296-3303.

[75] Poly, F., et al., Heterogeneity of a *Campylobacter jejuni* protein that is secreted through the flagellar filament. *Infection and Immunity*, 2007. 75: p. 3859-3867.

[76] Song, Y.C., et al., FlaC, a protein of *Campylobacter jejuni* TGH9011 (ATCC43431) secreted through the flagellar apparatus, binds epithelial cells and influences cell invasion. *Molecular Microbiology*, 2004. 53(2): p. 541-553.

[77] Neal-McKinney, J.M. and M.E. Konkel, The *Campylobacter jejuni* CiaC virulence protein is secreted from the flagellum and delivered to the cytosol of host cells. *Frontiers in Cellular and Infection Microbiology*, 2012. 2: p. 31.

[78] Malik-Kale, P., C.T. Parker, and M.E. Konkel, Culture of *Campylobacter jejuni* with sodium deoxycholate induces virulence gene expression. *Journal of Bacteriology*, 2008. 190: p. 2286-2297.

[79] Rivera-Amill, V., et al., Secretion of the virulence-associated *Campylobacter* invasion antigens from *Campylobacter jejuni* requires a stimulatory signal. *Journal of Infectious Diseases*, 2001. 183(11): p. 1607-1616.

[80] Buelow, D.R., et al., *Campylobacter jejuni* survival within human epithelial cells is enhanced by the secreted protein CiaI. *Molecular Microbiology,* 2011. 80: p. 1296-1312.

[81] Samuelson, D.R., et al., The *Campylobacter jejuni* CiaD effector protein activates MAP kinase signaling pathways and is required for the development of disease. *Cell Communication and Signaling*, 2013. 11: p. 79.

[82] Barrero-Tobon, A.M. and D.R. Hendrixson, Flagellar biosynthesis exerts temporal regulation of secretion of specific *Campylobacter jejuni* colonization and virulence determinants. *Molecular Microbiology*, 2014. 93(5): p. 957-74.

[83] Konkel, M.E., et al., The pathogenesis of *Campylobacter jejuni*-mediated enteritis. *Current Issues in Intesttinal Microbiology*, 2001. 2: p. 55-71.

[84] Raphael, B.H., et al., The *Campylobacter jejuni* response regulator, CbrR, modulates sodium deoxycholate resistance and chicken colonization. *Journal of Bacteriology*, 2005. 187(11): p. 3662-3670.

[85] Boehm, M., et al., Major host factors involved in epithelial cell invasion of *Campylobacter jejuni*: role of fibronectin, integrin beta1, FAK, Tiam-1, and DOCK180 in activating Rho GTPase Rac1. *Frontiers in Cellular and Infection Microbiology*, 2011. 1: p. 17.

[86] Cote, J.F. and K. Vuori, GEF what? Dock180 and related proteins help Rac to polarize cells in new ways. *Trends in Cell Biology*, 2007. 17(8): p. 383-93.

[87] Bouwman, L.I., P. Niewold, and J.P. van Putten, Basolateral invasion and trafficking of *Campylobacter jejuni* in polarized epithelial cells. *PLoS One*, 2013. 8(1): p. e54759.

[88] Konkel, M.E., et al., Invasion of epithelial cells by *Campylobacter jejuni* is independent of caveolae. *Cell Communication and Signaling*, 2013. 11: p. 100.

[89] Hu, L., et al., Enhanced microscopic definition of *Campylobacter jejuni* 81-176 adherence to, invasion of, translocation across, and exocytosis from polarized human intestinal Caco-2 cells. *Infection and Immunity*, 2008. 76(11): p. 5294-304.

[90] Kalischuk, L.D., G.D. Inglis, and A.G. Buret, *Campylobacter jejuni* induces transcellular translocation of commensal bacteria via lipid rafts. *Gut Pathogens*, 2009. 1(1): p. 2.

[91] Konkel, M.E., et al., Translocation of *Campylobacter jejuni* across human polarized epithelial-cell monolayer-cultures. *Journal of Infectious Diseases,* 1992. 166(2): p. 308-315.

[92] Monteville, M.R. and M.E. Konkel, Fibronectin-facilitated invasion of T84 eukaryotic cells by *Campylobacter jejuni* occurs preferentially at the basolateral cell surface. *Infection and Immunity*, 2002. 70(12): p. 6665-6671.

[93] Van Deun, K., et al., Butyrate protects Caco-2 cells from *Campylobacter jejuni* invasion and translocation. *British Journal of Nutrition*, 2008. 100(3): p. 480-4.

[94] Boehm, M., et al., Rapid paracellular transmigration of *Campylobacter jejuni* across polarized epithelial cells without affecting TER: role of proteolytic-active HtrA cleaving E-cadherin but not fibronectin. *Gut Pathogens,* 2012. 4(1): p. 3.

[95] Fry, B.N., et al., The *gal*E gene of *Campylobacter jejuni* is involved in lipopolysaccharide synthesis and virulence. *Infection and Immunity,* 2000. 68(5): p. 2594-2601.

[96] Marsden, G.L., et al., Creation of a large deletion mutant of *Campylobacter jejuni* reveals that the lipooligosaccharide gene cluster is not required for viability. *Journal of Bacteriology*, 2009. 191(7): p. 2392-9.

[97] Habib, I., et al., Correlation between genotypic diversity, lipooligosaccharide gene locus class variation, and caco-2 cell invasion potential of *Campylobacter jejuni* isolates from chicken meat and humans: contribution to virulotyping. *Applied and Environmental Microbiology,* 2009. 75(13): p. 4277-88.

[98] Louwen, R., et al., The sialylated lipooligosaccharide outer core in *Campylobacter jejuni* is an important determinant for epithelial cell invasion. *Infection and Immunity*, 2008. 76(10): p. 4431-4438.

[99] Mortensen, N.P., et al., Sialylation of *Campylobacter jejuni* lipo-oligosaccharides is associated with severe gastro-enteritis and reactive arthritis. *Microbes and Infection*, 2009. 11(12): p. 988-994.

[100] Guerry, P., et al., Phase variation of *Campylobacter jejuni* 81-176 lipooligosaccharide affects ganglioside mimicry and invasiveness in vitro. *Infection and Immunity*, 2002. 70(2): p. 787-93.

[101] Javed, M.A., et al., Cj1136 is required for lipooligosaccharide biosynthesis, hyperinvasion, and chick colonization by *Campylobacter jejuni*. *Infection and Immunity*, 2012. 80(7): p. 2361-70.

[102] Lertpiriyapong, K., et al., *Campylobacter jejuni* type VI secretion system: roles in adaptation to deoxycholic acid, host cell adherence, invasion, and *in vivo* colonization. *PLoS One*, 2012. 7(8): p. e42842.

[103] Bleumink-Pluym, N.M., et al., Identification of a functional type VI secretion system in *Campylobacter jejuni* conferring capsule polysaccharide sensitive cytotoxicity. *PLoS Pathogens*, 2013. 9(5): p. e1003393.

[104] Wassenaar, T.M., Toxin production by *Campylobacter* spp. *Clinical Microbiology Reviews*, 1997. 10(3): p. 466-&.

[105] Albert, M.J., et al., Identification of a *Campylobacter jejuni* protein that cross-reacts with cholera toxin. *Infection and Immunity*, 2007. 75(6): p. 3070-3.

[106] Gatsos, X., et al., Application of protein purification methods for the enrichment of a cytotoxin from *Campylobacter jejuni*. *BMC Microbiology,* 2012. 12: p. 303.

[107] Chien, C.C., et al., Identification of *cdt*B homologues and cytolethal distending toxin activity in enterohepatic *Helicobacter* spp. *Journal of Medical Microbiology*, 2000. 49(6): p. 525-34.

[108] Lara-Tejero, M. and J.E. Galan, CdtA, CdtB, and CdtC form a tripartite complex that is required for cytolethal distending toxin activity. *Infection and Immunity*, 2001. 69(7): p. 4358-65.

[109] Okuda, J., H. Kurazono, and Y. Takeda, Distribution of the cytolethal distending toxin A gene (*cdt*A) among species of *Shigella* and *Vibrio*, and cloning and sequencing of the *cdt* gene from *Shigella dysenteriae*. *Microbial Pathogenesis*, 1995. 18(3): p. 167-72.

[110] Peres, S.Y., et al., A new cytolethal distending toxin (CDT) from *Escherichia coli* producing CNF2 blocks HeLa cell division in G2/M phase. *Molecular Microbiology*, 1997. 24(5): p. 1095-107.

[111] Heywood, W., B. Henderson, and S.P. Nair, Cytolethal distending toxin: creating a gap in the cell cycle. *Journal of Medical Microbiology*, 2005. 54(Pt 3): p. 207-16.

[112] Hickey, T.E., G. Majam, and P. Guerry, Intracellular survival of Campylobacter jejuni in human monocytic cells and induction of apoptotic death by cytolethal distending toxin. *Infection and Immunity*, 2005. 73(8): p. 5194-5197.

[113] Zheng, J., et al., *Campylobacter*-induced interleukin-8 secretion in polarized human intestinal epithelial cells requires *Campylobacter*-secreted cytolethal distending toxin- and Toll-like receptor-mediated activation of NF-kappaB. *Infection and Immunity*, 2008. 76(10): p. 4498-508.

[114] Jain, D., et al., Differences in virulence attributes between cytolethal distending toxin positive and negative *Campylobacter* jejuni strains. *Journal of Medical Microbiology*, 2008. 57(Pt 3): p. 267-72.

[115] Biswas, D., et al., Effect of cytolethal distending toxin of *Campylobacter* jejuni on adhesion and internalization in cultured cells and in colonization of the chicken gut. *Avian Diseases*, 2006. 50(4): p. 586-593.

[116] Bang, D.D., et al., PCR detection of seven virulence and toxin genes of *Campylobacter jejuni* and *Campylobacter coli* isolates from Danish pigs and cattle and cytolethal distending toxin production of the isolates. *Journal of Applied Microbiology*, 2003. 94(6): p. 1003-14.

[117] Datta, S., H. Niwa, and K. Itoh, Prevalence of 11 pathogenic genes of *Campylobacter jejuni* by PCR in strains isolated from humans, poultry meat and broiler and bovine faeces. *Journal of Medical Microbiology*, 2003. 52(Pt 4): p. 345-8.

[118] Konkel, M.E., et al., Identification of the enteropathogens *Campylobacter jejuni* and *Campylobacter coli* based on the *cad*F virulence gene and its product. *Journal of Clinical Microbiology*, 1999. 37(3): p. 510-517.

[119] Ripabelli, G., et al., Prevalence of virulence-associated genes and cytolethal distending toxin production in *Campylobacter* spp. isolated in Italy. *Comparative Immunology Microbiology and Infectious Diseases*, 2010. 33(4): p. 355-64.

[120] Rozynek, E., et al., Prevalence of potential virulence markers in Polish *Campylobacter jejuni* and *Campylobacter coli* isolates obtained from hospitalized children and from chicken carcasses. *Journal of Medical Microbiology*, 2005. 54(Pt 7): p. 615-9.

[121] Talukder, K.A., et al., Prevalence of virulence genes and cytolethal distending toxin production in *Campylobacter jejuni* isolates from diarrheal patients in Bangladesh. *Journal of Clinical Microbiology*, 2008. 46(4): p. 1485-8.

[122] Krause-Gruszczynska, M., et al., Role of the small Rho GTPases Rac1 and Cdc42 in host cell invasion of *Campylobacter jejuni*. *Cellular Microbiology*, 2007. 9(10): p. 2431-44.

[123] Zautner, A.E., et al., Epidemiological association of *Campylobacter jejuni* groups with pathogenicity-associated genetic markers. *BMC Microbiology*, 2012. 12: p. 171.
[124] Dipineto, L., et al., *Campylobacter jejuni*, *Campylobacter coli*, and cytolethal distending toxin genes in laying hens. *Avian Diseases*, 2011. 55(1): p. 103-5.
[125] Gargiulo, A., et al., *Campylobacter jejuni*, *Campylobacter coli*, and cytolethal distending toxin (CDT) genes in common teals (*Anas crecca*). *Veterinary Microbiology*, 2011. 150(3-4): p. 401-4.
[126] Asakura, M., et al., Comparative analysis of cytolethal distending toxin (*cdt*) genes among *Campylobacter jejuni*, *C. coli* and *C. fetus* strains. *Microbial Pathogenesis*, 2007. 42(5-6): p. 174-83.
[127] Asakura, M., et al., Development of a cytolethal distending toxin (*cdt*) gene-based species-specific multiplex PCR assay for the detection and identification of *Campylobacter jejuni*, *Campylobacter coli* and *Campylobacter fetus*. *FEMS Immunology and Medical Microbiology*, 2008. 52(2): p. 260-6.
[128] Fernandes, M., et al., Study of cytolethal distending toxin (*cdt*) in *Campylobacter coli* using a multiplex polymerase chain reaction assay and its distribution among clinical and food strains. *Foodborne Pathogens Disease,* 2010. 7(1): p. 103-6.
[129] Kabir, S.M., et al., Evaluation of a cytolethal distending toxin (*cdt*) gene-based species-specific multiplex PCR assay for the identification of *Campylobacter* strains isolated from diarrheal patients in Japan. *Japanese Journal of Infectious Diseases*, 2011. 64(1): p. 19-27.
[130] Shiramaru, S., et al., A cytolethal distending toxin gene-based multiplex PCR assay for detection of *Campylobacter* spp. in stool specimens and comparison with culture method. *Journal of Veterinary Medical Science*, 2012. 74(7): p. 857-62.
[131] Heuvelink, A.E., et al., Two outbreaks of campylobacteriosis associated with the consumption of raw cows' milk. *International Journal of Food Microbiology*, 2009. 134(1-2): p. 70-4.
[132] Meinersmann, R.J., et al., Discrimination of *Campylobacter jejuni* isolates by *fla* gene sequencing. *Journal of Clinical Microbiology*, 1997. 35(11): p. 2810-4.
[133] Wassenaar, T.M., et al., Comparison of *Campylobacter fla*-SVR genotypes isolated from humans and poultry in three European regions. *Letters in Applied Microbiology*, 2009. 49(3): p. 388-95.

[134] Cossart P., Listeriology (1926-2007): the rise of a model pathogen. *Microbes Infection*, 2007. 9(10):1143-6.

[135] Ly K.T., and J.E. Casanova, Mechanisms of *Salmonella* entry into host cells. *Cellular Microbiology*, 2007. 9(9):2103-11.

[136] Sinha B., and M. Herrmann, Mechanism and consequences of invasion of endothelial cells by *Staphylococcus aureus*. *Thrombosis and Haemostasis,* 2005. 94(2):266-77.

[137] Velge P., et al., Multiplicity of *Salmonella* entry mechanisms, a new paradigm for *Salmonella pathogenesis*. *Microbiology Open,* 2012. 1(3):243-58.

[138] Sinha B., and M. Fraunholz, *Staphylococcus aureus* host cell invasion and post-invasion events. *International Journal of Medical Microbiology*, 2010. 300(2-3):170-5.

[139] Pizarro-Cerdá J., A. Kühbacher, and P. Cossart. Entry of *Listeria monocytogenes* in mammalian epithelial cells: an updated view. *Cold Spring Harbor Perspectives in Medicine*, 2012. 1;2(11).

In: Campylobacter Infections
Editor: Brittany A. Bertucci

ISBN: 978-1-63463-858-6

Chapter 2

Campylobacter Infections: Epidemiology, Diagnosis, Control and Prevention

Soumaya Messaoudi and Michel Federighi*
Lunam, Oniris, Alim-SCAN research department, SECALIM
Nantes, France

Abstract

Campylobacter is now considered as a major agent of bacteriological foodborne diseases. This microorganism is capable to cause a very large number of cases of digestive campylobacteriosis, worldwide. Its high intestinal carriage by several livestock (poultry, swine, bovine, ovine…) is the reason why these animals are primary reservoirs of this microorganism. The quantitative importance of these primary reservoirs leads to its introduction into various habitats and to a contamination of foods, which can take place at any stage of the food production. After contamination, its survival and its ability to cause disease after ingestion of a low minimum infective dose do the rest. The disease is present in all parts of the world, preferably in summer, and in all populations, but with peaks for the age groups 0-5 years, 20-30 years and above 60 years. Medical treatment may be conventional, often symptomatic, sometimes associated with the use of antibiotics in some severe cases. The

* Author for correspondance : michel.federighi@oniris-nantes.fr.

development of a vaccine strategy is difficult even if there have been significant advances in recent years in the field. However, digestive campylobacteriosis transmitted by foods are not unavoidable because there are, at all stages of the food chain, many truly effective control measures to reduce the contamination of foods by Campylobacter. Their effective implementation and coordination in an integrated approach of hygiene management, will reduce the incidence of this disease.

1. Introduction

Currently best known as one of the main agents involved in foodborne disease, *Campylobacter* have historically been first associated with animal health problems. The first microscopic observation of these microorganisms is carried out by Escherich in Germany in 1886 in samples of children diarrhea. Then McFadyean and Stockman were the first to isolate a microaerophilic spiral bacterium called "vibrion" in animal samples. From that date, "vibrion" were regularly isolated in abortion problems or diarrhea in sheep, cattle and pigs. In 1946, Levy describes an outbreak of gastroenteritis in a prison in Illinois involving a microaerophilic spiral bacterium, presumably the current *Campylobacter jejuni*. This is probably the first description of a digestive foodborne campylobacteriosis (Federighi 1999a). Since the creation of genus *Campylobacter* by Sebald et Véron in 1963, the ID card of *Campylobacter* is well known (Table 1).

Table 1. ID card of *Campylobacter*

Kingdom	Eubacteria
Phylum	Proteobacteria
Class	Epsilonproteobacteria
Order	Campylobacterales
Family	*Campylobacteraceae* (with Arcobacter and Sulfurospirillum)
Genus	*Campylobacter*

Today, the genus *Campylobacter* brings together a very diverse variety of species with very diverse habitats, such as the oral cavity of humans (*C. concisus, C. curvus* or *C. showae*), the preputial cavity of bulls (*C. fetus subsp. venerealis* or *C. sputorum subsp. bubulus*) or gastrointestinal tract of many warm-blooded animals (*C. jejuni, C. coli, C. lari*) (Table 2). Of these species, one is largely predominant over others in its involvement in the problems of food safety: *Campylobacter jejuni*. It should be noted that despite this dominance, other species present an interest in the area of food safety: *C. fetus subsp. fetus*, *C. coli, C. upsaliensis* and *C. lari* mainly. Furthermore, the distinction between *C. jejuni subsp. doylei* and *C. jejuni subsp. jejuni* is rarely made by the authors, who use the expression *C. jejuni* to talk indistinctly of these two subspecies. We will do the same in the rest of this chapter, which will focus on this species.

Table 2. Genus *Campylobacter*: species and sub-species

Species	Sub-species
Campylobacter avium	
Campylobacter canadensis	
Campylobacter coli	
Campylobacter concisus	
Campylobacter cuniculorum	
Campylobacter curvus	
Campylobacter fetus	*C. fetus* subsp. *venerealis*
	C. fetus subsp. *fetus*
Campylobacter gracilis	
Campylobacter helveticus	
Campylobacter hominis	
Campylobacter hyointestinalis	*C. hyointestinalis* subsp. *hyointestinalis*
	C. hyointestinalis subsp. *lawsonii*
Campylobacter insulaenigrae	
Campylobacter jejuni	*C. jejuni* subsp. *doylei*
	C. jejuni subsp. *jejuni*
Campylobacter lanienae	
Campylobacter lari	*C. lari* subsp. *concheus*
	C. lari subsp. *lari*
Campylobacter mucosalis	
Campylobacter peloridis	
Campylobacter rectus	
Campylobacter showae	
Campylobacter sputorum	*C. sputorum* biovar Sputorum
	C. sputorum biovar Faecalis
	C. sputorum biovar Paraureolyticus
Campylobacter subantarcticus	
Campylobacter upsaliensis	
Campylobacter ureolyticus	
Campylobacter volucris	

2. Generalities

Campylobacter jejuni is a gram-negative bacillus of 0.2 to 0.5 μm in diameter and 1-8 μm in length. It's in the shape of « S », helical or spiral. It has one or more undulations and generally has a single polar flagellum. This structure gives to the microorganism a very high mobility, easily observable under the microscope (corkscrew-like motion). *Campylobacter jejuni* does not form a spore. After several days of culture appear frequently rounded shapes or coccoides bodies (0.5 μm diameter). It seems that we can assimilate them into degenerative forms (Federighi et al. 1998).

The main reservoir of *C. jejuni* is represented by animals (wild, domestic livestock or pets)), with an intestinal carriage. Among these animals it is accepted that birds are the main reservoir in terms of percentage of infected animals and of quantitative importance of intestinal carriage. This predominance of birds should not make us forget, or neglect, other known reservoirs represented by others domestic livestock: cattle, pigs and sheep, as well as pets (cats and dogs).

Campylobacter jejuni is considered a microaerophilic microorganism, growth occurs in the presence of an oxygen-depleted atmosphere (between 5 and 10%). In air, the accumulation of peroxides in the cell inhibits growth. For optimum performance, the culture media should contain compounds for trapping toxic elements and / or promoting the synthesis of detoxifying enzymes by *C. jejuni* (sodium pyruvate, thioglycolate, blood, charcoal...).

Many authors believe that *Campylobacter jejuni* is more capnophilic than microaerophilic (i.e it will require an enriched CO_2 atmosphere for growth (usually 10%)). The gas mixture generally used for its culture is (O_2 = 5% CO_2 = 10% N_2 = 85%)(Table 3).

Table 3. Main factors for *Campylobacter jejuni* growth

	OPTIMUM	INHIBITION
Temperature	37 à 41,5°C	< 30°C ou >45°C
pH	6,5 - 7,5	< 4,7 ou >8,2
O_2	5 - 10%	0% ou > 15-19%
CO_2	10%	/
a_w	0,997	< 0,987
NaCl	0,5%	1,5%

All *Campylobacter* species can grow at 37 ° C, these are real mesophilic. *C. jejuni* can grow in a temperature range from 30 ° C to 45 ° C but not at 25 ° C, which differentiates it from some other species of *Campylobacter*. The optimum pH range for growth is 6.5 to 7.5. Finally, the presence of 0.5% sodium chloride (NaCl) in the growth medium is recommended, while concentrations above 1.5% tend to inhibit its growth. In Petri dishes, colonies usually appear after 24 to 48 hours. In some cases, it is necessary to wait five days to see the colonies. On blood agar plates, there is no lysis. Since the 80s there has been a lot of development of different culture media for *Campylobacter*. In recent years chromogenic agars are appeared. It's a real progress for the routine analysis of *Campylobacter* (Remize et al. 2013).

3. Digestive Human Campylobacteriosis

As we have seen before, several species of *Campylobacter* are capable to cause to man a disease called digestive campylobacteriosis: namely *C. jejuni*, *C. coli*, *C. lari* and *C. upsaliensis*. The transmission, from reservoir to man, of *Campylobacter* cells is direct or indirect. Handling animals carrying *Campylobacter* will contaminate the hands, which are then brought to the mouth: this is the direct transmission. The indirect way is the consumption of food or water contaminated with *Campylobacter* cells. The main risk factors for direct transmission are: contact with domestic animals (poultry, cattle, pigs, sheep), diarrheic kittens or puppies, as well as ingestion of contaminated recreational water. However, this remains a relatively rare event. Indirect transmission is much more common since it will be the cause of more than 80% of digestive human campylobacteriosis (Alter and Scherer, 2006).

3.1. Clinical Aspects of Human Campylobacteriosis

The clinical picture of the digestive campylobacteriosis is not pathognomonic and can sometimes be confused with that caused by other enteric pathogens. This is an acute enteritis may be complicated by bacteremia, secondary locations and post-infective syndrome. The incubation period lasts an average of 3.2 days (8 hours minimum, maximum 8 days). It is generally described a diarrhea (85% of cases), abdominal pain, bloody stools, fever and sometimes nausea and vomiting. In the majority of cases (80%), the disease is self-limiting within a week, but the bacterium persists in the stool for several weeks (Table 4).

In patients, the expression of various clinical pictures put on a path of at least three distinct pathogenic mechanisms: (i) it may be a simple secretory diarrhea, involving adhesion and colonization with synthesis of enterotoxins; (ii) diarrhea may be bloody or mucous indicating proliferation (after penetration) of the bacteria in the intestinal mucosa, and inflammatory response; (iii) the existence of extra-intestinal complications show that the bacteria pass through or between enterocytes, it is taken up by the circulatory torrents to reach specific targets.

Table 4. Main characteristics of digestive campylobacteriosis

Mean duration of the prodomal phase	Mean duration of symptomatic phase	Main symptoms Median frequency of symptom % (Range)
3.2 days (8h to 8d)	3 to 4 days	• Diarrhea: 85 % (52 - 100) • Abdominal pain : 79% (56 - 99) • Blood in feces: 15% (0.5 – 32) • Fever: 50 % (6 – 75) • Headache: 41% (6 – 69) • Vomiting: 15 % (1 – 42) **Acute self-limiting enteritis in 80% of cases**
Duration of the infectious period	**Frequency (%) of complications (including lethality)**	
Mean : 37.6 days Max. : 69 days	• Bacteriema et septicemia : <1% • Guillain-Barré syndrome : 0.1% • Lethality : <0.1% des cas	

Colonization of the Gastrointestinal Tract

During digestive campylobacteriosis, enumeration of *Campylobacter* in stool samples can reveal 10^6 to 10^9 cells per gram, which clearly indicates that there is colonization of the gastrointestinal tract. In the literature, there is some consensus that intestinal colonization is done according to a standard scheme: (i) adhesion to the surface mucus, (ii) penetration of the mucus and, (iii) Association / adhesion to intestinal epithelial cells. For *Campylobacter*, colonization seems easier because, firstly, there are optimal conditions for its growth in the intestine: high temperature (37 ° to 39 ° C) and microaerophilic conditions. In this regard, it has been shown that the adherence factor CBF1 (Campylobacter Binding Factor) plays a key role for optimal growth under these conditions (Müller et al. 2007). Secondly, intrinsic factors like resistance to bile salts, its morphology and mobility, as well as its positive chemotaxis for mucus provide to *Campylobacter* a selective advantage on the commensal flora.

Adherence to Intestinal Cells

The main target for *Campylobacter* adherence to intestinal cells seems to be the brush border of the enterocytes or goblet cells. Adherence is reversible, multifactorial and motility-dependent. Several adhesins (real or putative) have been described, among them CADF (Campylobacter adhesion to Fibronectin) and CBF1 play an important role. However, it seems established that *C. jejuni* uses several adherence mechanisms, specific or not. Of these, the flagellum, apart from its role in motility and adhesion, plays a role in the secretion of non-flagellar proteins involved in the invasion of enterocytes (i.e., Cia, Campylobacter Invasion Antigen) (Guerry, 2007).

Invasion of Intestinal Cells

The inflammatory tissue lesions, the presence of blood and leukocytes in the diarrheal stools during the campylobacteriosis evoke a *Shigella spp.* dysentery or *Entamoeba histolytica*, invasive microorganisms. Indeed, the property to invade epithelial cells has been demonstrated *in vitro* for some *Campylobacter* strains in cell cultures models (Caco-2 and INT 407) (Federighi, 2005). In addition, *Campylobacter* can pass the intestinal barrier (named translocation). The translocation of *C. jejuni* can be done through (transcellular route) or between (paracellular route) the epithelial cells and involves the synthesis of proteins Cia. A reorganization of the cytoskeleton of intestinal cells has been shown in response to signal adherence of *C. jejuni*. The CDT (Cytolethal Distending Toxin), secreted by *Campylobacter jejuni*, could be one of those signals. It should be noted that other studies conducted in Caco-2 cells showed internalization of *C. jejuni* without rearrangement of the cytoskeleton of these cells, defending the hypothesis of a passive internalization (Konkel et al. 2000). After penetration into cells, *C. jejuni* can survive in vacuoles and prevent the phagosome-lysosome fusion to avoid phagocytosis and can induce the production of interleukin-8 (pro-inflammatory response) or apoptosis of host cells (Young et al. 2007).

Others Factors Involved in Virulence

Several factors are regularly cited as playing a role in the pathogenicity of *Campylobacter*:

- The capsule involved in resistance to the bactericidal effect of serum and adhesion,
- The SODB (superoxide dismutase) important in resistance to macrophages,
- The synthesis of siderophores involved for *in situ* capture of iron, necessary for the survival,
- Or the CDT (Cytolethal Distending Toxin) capable of producing, *in vitro*, cell distension of different cell lines (CHO, Vero, Hela and Hep2).

3.2. Dose Response Relationship

The dose / response relationship for *Campylobacter* is unclear. Obviously, it is multifactorial and depends on: (i) the sensitivity of the host, (ii) the characteristics of ingested contaminated food (protective effect against gastric acidity), (iii) the virulence of ingested strains and, (iv) the immune status of the host vis-à-vis *Campylobacter*.

A single experiment has clarified the effect dose / response for *C. jejuni* (Black et al. 1988). This consisted of the ingestion of two strains, by human volunteers. Both strains were ingested in milk or a solution of baking soda in doses ranging from $8x10^2$ to $2x10^9$ CFU (Colony Forming Unit). Increasing the dose is clearly associated with an increase in infection rates but not necessarily with the onset of symptoms. In this experiment, the main target for *Campylobacter* colonization seems to be the colon, although this microorganism is also able to colonize the small intestine. Finally, the authors claimed that, according to their study and in natural conditions, low doses of *Campylobacter* could trigger the disease. An epidemic in Canada has confirmed this hypothesis. Indeed, the enumeration of *Campylobacter* in pieces of meat involved in this epidemic, revealed the presence of only 460 cells per 120 grams of meat (Federighi, 1999a).

3.3. Medical Treatment

Campylobacter jejuni enteritis generally has a good prognosis, even with only symptomatic treatment. In case of absence of antibiotherapy, excretion of the microorganism in the stools lasts longer. Usually, antibiotherapy is reserved for patients with severe clinical picture (persistent diarrhea, significant loss of weight, bloody diarrhea...) or a serious underlying disease (HIV +, agammaglobulinemia ...). Macrolids, in particular Erythromycin, are often the first choice treatment due to its narrow spectrum. Fluoroquinolones such as ciprofloxacin were also used in digestive campylobacteriosis. They may also be used in dual therapy (fluoroquinolone + Gentamicin). In some severe cases of dehydration, parenteral rehydration is required. The research on the development of a vaccine is still current. However, the development of whole-cell vaccines is difficult in front of the risks of complications (Guillain-Barré syndrome), and the choice of an ideal antigenic protein for the production of a vaccine is not yet decided. In conclusion, it should be noted that the treatment in case of Guillain-Barré syndrome is plasmapheresis.

3.4. Transmission to Man by Foods

3.4.1. Prevalence of Campylobacter in Foods

Epidemics of campylobacteriosis are rare, most cases are sporadic cases. In the absence of investigations into these sporadic cases, there is therefore an important loss of informations about the foods causing these cases. Under these conditions, the use of existing case-control studies is very helpful. They allow to regularly highlighting the role of chicken meat (Doorduyn et al. 2010) (Table 5). This fact was confirmed by a study conducted in Belgium during the dioxin crisis, which showed that the number of campylobacteriosis declined by 40% during the withdrawal from sale of poultry (Vellinga and Van Loock, 2002).

Numerous studies of survey of thermotolerant *Campylobacter* in food have been published for nearly thirty years. This allows, today, to have a good representation of the prevalence of *Campylobacter* in different foods. Thus, meat and offal of chicken, turkey or duck have very high positive rate between 30 and 100%, according to the studies. Once the products have been processed, the prevalence is generally lower. Indeed, the transformation process applied may have a very important effect on the presence of *Campylobacter* in foods. For example, processes such as salting, drying and / or smoking significantly reduce the prevalence of *Campylobacter* in duck meat (Remize et al. 2013). It should be noted, finally, that for the poultry industry, eggs and egg products are not usually considered as products carrying *Campylobacter*.

Red meats (meat and offal) are described with varying prevalences across studies, but generally lower than those of poultry meat. It is recognized that the red meat contamination occurs at the slaughterhouse. When the slaughter process is totally « under control », the prevalence of *Campylobacter* on meat or carcasses is limited (usually 0-10%). This is clear for pork, it is more difficult to be so positive for sheep and cattle where some studies report high rates of positive (up to 70%) on meat and offal collected in store. It should be noted that for red meat, it is accepted that offals have comparable prevalence than meat (Jacobs-Reitsma et al. 2008).

For milk and dairy products, the scientific literature tells us that these are not products which have a high prevalence for *Campylobacter*. In fact, many studies show very low rates of positive for raw milk (cows or goats)(from 0% to a maximum of 10%) (Federighi, 2005, Jacobs-Reitsma et al. 2008). For example, none *Campylobacter* has been isolated after analysis of 140 samples of raw milk cheeses by ISO 10272 method (Federighi et al. (1999b)). Yogurt and butter (especially salted) are not known to be contaminated by *Campylobacter*. However, an outbreak of campylobacteriosis associated with butter "Maître d'hôtel" (butter + garlic + parsley) in a restaurant was described by Zhao et al. (Cited by Jacobs -Reitma et al. 2008).

Table 5. Examples of case-control studies (adapted from Federighi (2007))

Country	Nb of cases	Nb of controls	Main risk factors
USA (Washington)	218	526	Consumption of poorly cooked chicken, raw fish and shellfish
USA	45	45	Consumption of chicken. Contact with a cat
Norway	52	103	Consumption of chicken bought raw and sausages cooked on a barbecue
New Zealand	100	100	Consumption of chicken outside the home and untreated water
Switzerland	167	282	Overseas travel. Consumption of chicken
United Kingdom	598	598	Handling of raw meat. Contact with a diarrheic pet. Consumption of untreated water
New Zealand	621	621	Consumption of chicken undercooked or in a restaurant. Overseas travel. Use of rain water. Consumption of raw milk. Contact with animals
Sweden	101	198	Consumption of raw milk. Consumption of chicken and pork. Food cooked on a barbecue
USA (Hawaï)	211	211	Consumption of chicken outside the home. Ingestion of antibiotics
Netherland	1315	3409	Consumption of undercooked chicken, Contact with pets. Taking medication (protom pump inhibitor)
Denmark	282	319	Consumption of undercooked chicken, red meat cooked on a barbecue, grapes and raw milk. Overseas travel
Norway	212	422	Consumption of untreated water, meat cooked on a barbecue and chicken bought raw. Contact with animals. Consumption of poorly cooked pork
USA	1316	1316	Consumption of chicken outside the home and red meat prepared in a restaurant. Contact with animal feces or young pets

Water has been described as a vector for the transmission of *Campylobacter*. Outbreaks were caused by contaminated water due to inadequate control of treatment and / or extreme weather events leading to recontamination of the water after treatment network.

Evans et al. (2003) indicated that the bottled water could be a risk factor for campylobacteriosis.

However, no *Campylobacter* could be isolated from the analysis of 200 bottles (50 cl) according to ISO 17995 method (Federighi, unpublished data). However, the survival of the organism in an artificially contaminated mineral water is possible for several days (Guillou et al. 2003).

Campylobacter prevalence in other foods has been established by several studies. It shows that vegetables are usually very weakly positive: 1-3% for 1560 samples analyzed by Park and Sanders (1992) and 0.5% (400 samples of vegetables) for Federighi et al. (1999b). Conversely, Chai et al. (2007) describe positive rate of 29-67% for raw vegetables used in the preparation of salads in Malaysia.

Implicated in the late 80s, fungi do not appear to be so-called "at risk" in other studies (Jacobs-Reitsma et al. 2008).

Finally, we must mention bivalve molluscs (oysters, mussels, cockles...) involved in several sporadic cases or in epidemics (Abeyta et al. 1993). In oysters, some authors (cited by Jacobs-Reitsma et al. 2008) indicate high positive rate (14-67%), other authors show very low rate (0.5%) (Federighi et al. (1997)). It is important to note that (i) *Campylobacter lari* is often isolated in these products, (ii) "hot" months (March-November for the northern hemisphere) and (iii) the location of parks shellfish beds near potentially contaminated sources (sewage effluents, farmland runoff) are more favorable to contamination with *Campylobacter* (Jacobs-Reitsma et al. 2008).

3.4.2. Survey in Foods

Detection of *Campylobacter spp.* in foods can be done in different circumstances, it may be regulatory or voluntary. In all cases, it is recommended to use the standard method appeared in the 90s (revised in 2006), namely the ISO 10272-1 which the different steps are presented in the table 6 below.

The 2006 revision also allowed the development of a standard (ISO / TS 10272-2) on the enumeration of *Campylobacter*. It is clear from reading this table that the search for thermotolerant *Campylobacter* in food is time consuming, requiring an enrichment period never inferior than one day and cultures and subcultures also requiring several days.

Table 6. Different steps of the ISO 10272 norm: "detection of thermophilics *Campylobacter* in foods" (revised version (2006))

Sample	*X grams (e.g 10g or 25g) or X mL*		
Homogenization & ten-fold dilution	*9X mL of nutrient broth*		
Enrichment	*Bolton method*	*Preston method*	*Park & Sanders method*
	Incubation in microaerophilic atmosphere at 37°C for 4h to 6h	*Incubation in microaerophilic atmosphere at 41,5°C (18h)*	*Addition of the « antibiotic A » solution and incubation in microaerophilic atmosphere at 32 ° C for 4 h*
	Incubation in microaerophilic atmosphere at 41.5°C for 44h (±4h)		*Addition of the « antibiotic B » solution and incubation in microaerophilic atmosphere at 37°C for 4h*
			Incubation in microaerophilic atmosphere at 41,5°C for 40h
Isolation and incubation	*Isolation on two selective agars – Incubation for 24 to 48h in microaerophilic atmosphere*		
	mCCDA agar (modified Charcoal Cefoperazone Deoxycholate Agar) *free choice for the second selective agar (including chromogenic agars)*		
Confirmation	Identification tests made on 5 presomptive colonies		

The Park & Sanders method is the most effective method for the detection of *Campylobacter* cells that are assumed stressed and / or damaged by the transformation process (freezing, heating, salting, drying...), but it's very fastidious. Preston method is the simplest to use, it takes less time, but it is less effective than the Park & Sanders method (Federighi et al. 1999b). Regarding the detection of *Campylobacter* on chicken carcasses, an aliquot of 10g of neck skin remains the preferred sampling strategy (Baré *et al.* 2013). The Bolton method appeared in the revised version of the standard, in 2006. It's a compromise between the two others methods. Finally, in 2005, appeared a method for the detection and enumeration of *Campylobacter* in water (ISO 17995 standard).

3.5. Epidemiology

Campylobacter is today in the role of a "leader" of infectious foodborne diseases. In the United States each year, the number of Campylobacter infections is around 2,4 millions, higher than Salmonella infections (Friedman et al. 2000).

In Europe (25 countries), a total of 183,961 confirmed cases of campylobacteriosis were recorded in 2004. Since then, the number of confirmed cases has increased steadily to reach, for example, 212,000 confirmed cases in 2012 (EFSA, 2012 Annual Report). In 2013, that number reached 220 000 confirmed cases (incidence: 48.2 / 100 000 inhabitant) for 25 reporting countries (EFSA, 2013 Annual Report). In all cases, *C. jejuni* is the dominant species (81 to 94% of cases) in Campylobacter infections. This microorganism is the most common cause of infectious foodborne illness in industrialized countries. Sporadic cases are the main form of expression of Campylobacter infections.

Contact with diarrheic pets (puppies and kittens) or domestic (farm animals) infected, travels abroad (developing countries), contact with raw meat are also risk factors for acquisition of Campylobacter infections. The transmission from man to man is rare. Several studies show that the risk factors for common source outbreaks are not quite the same as risk factors for sporadic infections.

Large and foodborne common source outbreaks are rare. In the United States they represent less than 1% of foodborne outbreaks reported. Water and raw milk are the main sources of contamination identified during major epidemics in the United States and the countries of Northern Europe (Table 7).

In France, an outbreak linked to the consumption of tap water contaminated by several pathogenic bacteria including *Campylobacter coli*, occurred in 2000. This outbreak has affected about 2,600 people (62 confirmed cases) of the same town (Gallay et al. 2006). There are various other food sources capable to cause epidemics; it seems to be due to a transfer of contamination (cross contamination) during food preparation, with contaminated poultry as the main source. For some authors, the lack of proper hand washing, poor hygiene practices when cooking and a low level of information and knowledge on domestic hygiene are the main risk factors that apply to New Zealand's world record of notifications of campylobacteriosis per capita (Al-Sakkaf, 2012). For this author, enhancing hygiene in food preparation at home and outside the home is a priority action for the coming years in the fight against digestive foodborne campylobacteriosis.

Table 7. Examples of common source epidemics for *Campylobacter* (adapted from Silva *et al.* (2011))

Country	Number of cases	Food involved in the transmission	Year
USA (California)	12	Raw milk	1984
France	62	Tap water	2000
Denmark	79	Chicken salad	2005
Australia	11	Chicken	2005
Spain	81	Sour cream	2005
Norway	105	Tap water	2007
Canada	225	Unknow	2007
USA	5	Raw milk	2008
Greece	27	Tap water	2009
United Kingdom	24	Chicken (offals)	2010

4. Control Measure – Good Hygienic Practices

There is no proliferation of *Campylobacter* in foods, so there exist two main approaches to control *Campylobacter jejuni* in food industry:

- prevention of contamination in breeding, food industries, during transport and in food preparation inside or outside home;
- complete or sufficient destruction of *Campylobacter jejuni* in foods by physical or chemical methods.

4.1. Preventive Approach

The sources of *Campylobacter* contamination are numerous and it is therefore essential to control all possible entry points of bacteria all along the food production chain.

To avoid any proliferation in water supply network, installations must be both well designed and well maintained. Water treatment must be suitable for this type of contamination and its efficacy should be tested regularly.

The animal reservoir, notably the avian reservoir, being the principal source of contamination, measures must be taken right from breeding to prevent or minimize colonization of domestic livestock.

Breeding is an important link for this control because it has several opportunities to intervene (Messaoudi et al. 2013). Thus, good hygienic practices and biosecurity measures can be a strategy to prevent colonization of animals by *Campylobacter* (procedures of disinfection between every batches, steady change of clothes, disinfecting hands and boots, treatment of drinking water, the fight against the introduction of macro-pests in henhouses, installation of mosquito nets...). This interest is strengthened by the development of indirect measures, additional to good practices, to reduce the intestinal carriage of *Campylobacter* in poultry. These strategies can be of two types:

- Global and preventive, intervening early in the lives of animals and intended to reduce or even to prevent colonization of animals by *Campylobacter*. Include: vaccination, genetic selection and the use of prebiotics and probiotics.
- More focused on *Campylobacter* and a few days before slaughter in order to provide to slaughter animals whose the intestinal carriage of *Campylobacter* is reduced. These include: the use of food additives, bacteriophage and bacteriocins.

Specific measures to slaughterhouses have been described in the development of HACCP systems (Hazard Analysis Critical Control Point). They are based on the implementation of prerequisite programs able to maintain at all times a good hygienic environment of production. Equipment and surfaces should be regularly disinfected and machine maintenance performed regularly. It is important to ensure that the different scalding and cooling procedures are well respected. Defeathering is an operation that deserves a particular attention, such as evisceration. Throughout the chain, personnel, properly trained, should follow good hygienic practices of slaughtering and systematically eliminate substandard carcasses. The transporters and distributors must take care to employ the correct storage conditions and never to put in contact raw poultry meat with other non-contamined foods. If this is necessary, it is strongly recommended to use protective films. Finally, the last precautions concern the preparation of meals inside or outside the home. It is essential to clean the refrigerator regularly and to separate raw meat from other foods. Utensils used for cutting meat should be systematically washed before any other use. Avoid consuming raw milk or untreated water, and cook meat to a temperature above 65 ° C in all parts of the meat. A study of cross-contamination in kitchens has shown it advisable to reserve certain working areas specifically for poultry (cutting board for example) and recommends to increase the level of hygiene in kitchens at home (Kusumaningrum *et al.* 2004). Moreover, the presence of pets (dogs, cats, birds) in the house requires increased vigilance, especially when they (or their accessories) are handled (litter, bowls, feeders...).

4.2. Destruction of *Campylobacter* in Foods

4.2.1. Physical Treatments

- Temperature

Campylobacter are very sensitive to high temperatures. Today we can say that heat treatments are an excellent control measure of this hazard. Indeed, whatever the size of the population and the nature of the food matrix (liquid or solid), the application, at all points of the volume of the food, of a temperature above 65 ° C, destroyed *Campylobacter* in a few minutes (Federighi, 1999a) (Table 8).

Table 8. D values for *Campylobacter jejuni* (adapted from Federighi, 1999a)

Liquid media			
	Temperature (°C)	*D value (min)*	*Nb of tested strains*
Phosphate buffer	58	0,24 – 0,28	3
Milk	53	1 – 2,2	3
	56	0,3 – 0,9	2
	60	0,2 – 0,3	3

Solid media			
	Temperature (°C)	*D value (min)*	
Chicken	50	8,7 – 9,2	5
	55	2,12 – 2,25	5
	58	0,7 – 0,9	5
Beef	50	6,28 (sliced meat)	2
	56	0,96	2
	58	0,35	8
Lamb	56	1,23	2
	60	0,26	2

At temperatures of freezing (-20°C) and refrigeration (0 to 10°C) the survival remains significant. A study performed on chicken meat showed that refrigeration at 4°C led to a reduction of the population of 0.31 to 0.81 log10 CFU/g in 3 to 7 days and freezing to a reduction of 0.56 to 3.39 log10 CFU/g in 2 weeks (Bhaduri & Cottrell, 2004). During refrigeration, increasing the air speed diminished the survival of *Campylobacter* in the product while increasing its desiccation, although the texture of chicken skin seemed to protect the bacteria.

- Ionization

Campylobacter are also highly sensitive to ionizing radiation. The irradiation parameters necessary for their inactivation are largely inferior to those required to eliminate other enteropathogens like *Salmonella* or *E. coli.* Thus, doses of less than or equal to 1 kGy are quite sufficient to significantly reduce the number of viable cells and may be recommended to prevent infection by *Campylobacter* (Lewis et al. 2002).

- UltraViolets Radiation

Use of U.V. lamps for germicide applications in the purification of water has been known for a long time. In 1987 Butler et al. investigated the sensitivity of *C. jejuni* to U.V. radiation at 254 nm. This microbe appeared to be much more sensitive to ultraviolet radiation as compared to *E. coli* (1.8 versus 5 mws/cm^2) and they concluded that commercially available U.V. lamps could easily inactivate *C. jejuni*. Few works are devoted to treatment of *Campylobacter* with Intense Pulsed Light (Elmnasser et al. 2007). It appears that these new treatments are very effective *in vitro*, allowing several decimal reductions. However, the bacterial destruction at the surface of food is more disappointing (about 1 decimal reduction) and very dependent on the exposure of microorganisms to the light (shadow effect) (Murdoch et al. 2010, Haughton et al. 2012).

- Microwaves

Choi et al. (1993) studied the survival of *C. jejuni* in milk after microwave treatment (1380 watts). Three minutes of heating (temperature reached 71.1°C) were sufficient to definitively eliminate all *C. jejuni* cells, whereas eight minutes were required for *Yersinia enterocolitica*. One minute of heating reduced the population of *C. jejuni* by more than 5 logs.

- High Hydrostatic Pressure

Some recent but still rare studies have clearly shown that treatments of relatively short duration (10 min) at pressures of less than 400 MPa are sufficient to obtain an important decimal reduction of the population, the effect increasing with increasing pressure (Solomon & Hoover, 2004). This result was confirmed by Bièche *et al.* (2009) showed that, on two strains of *C. jejuni*, 400 MPa for 10 min at 20°C may produce more than 7 logarithmic reductions at pH 5.6 or 7. As in the case of other physical methods, a protective role of the food with respect to the treatment has been demonstrated, as compared to treatment in artificial media (buffers or broths) (Martinez-Rodriguez and Mackey 2005).

4.2.2. Chemical Treatment – Modified Atmosphere

The pH of most products susceptible harboring *Campylobacter* is compatible with survival of this microorganism, whereas it survives poorly when the pH lies below 4 or above 9. The foods and drinks most frequently incriminated in cases of campylobacteriosis (meat, milk, water) thus have a pH compatible with survival of the bacteria. On the contrary, an important bacteriostatic effect is observed at pH values of less than 4, particularly when the drop in pH is due to the presence of organic acids. Salting or addition of ascorbic acid likewise diminishes the survival of *Campylobacter*. Purification of water by treatment with chlorine enables rapid destruction of *Campylobacter*. Chlorine is also used in the United States to clean chicken carcasses and thereby permits partial reduction of the population (0.5 $\log_{10}$ CFU/ml after cleaning with water containing 25-35 ppm chlorine) (Bashor et al. 2004). Similarly, cleaning of carcasses by passage through a bath containing trisodium phosphate allows in an important decrease in the level of contamination (by about 2 logs, see below). Addition of ascorbic acid to a nutritive medium (5 mmol/L) has a bactericidal effect on *C. jejuni* at 42°C and according to the work of Juven et al. (1988), this effect could be extended to meat. These authors inoculated two batches of turkey meat with *C. jejuni* and stored them at +5°C for 7 weeks. As of the second week, the samples supplemented with 5 mmol/kg ascorbic acid gave a culturable cell count 2 logs lower than that of non-supplemented samples.

In the air, the survival of *Campylobacter* is limited. Conversely, the conditioning of food products under vacuum or in an atmosphere enriched in CO_2 does not seem to lead to any notable decrease in the survival of the bacteria (Dykes & Moorhead, 2001).

4.2.3. Miscellaneous

Bacteriocins

In 1992 Schoeni and Doyle isolated bacteria colonizing the cecum of white leghorn laying hens, which are *C. jejuni* free. Nine strains were found to produce metabolites against *Campylobacter* (colicins). In 2006, Stern et al. demonstrated the efficacy of a bacteriocin produced by a strain of *Lactobacillus salivarius* in reducing the carriage of *Campylobacter* by chickens. More recently, Messaoudi et al. have isolated a new strain of *Lactobacillus salivarius*, which has an anti-Campylobacter activity. A novel peptide: salivaricin SMXD51 is responsible for this activity (Messaoudi et al. 2012).

Spices & Essential Oils

The effects of oregano, sage and cloves on *C. jejuni* have been studied at different temperatures. Globally, these three substances at concentrations of 0.5 % have an inhibitory action on *C. jejuni* during the first 16 hours of conservation (Deibel and Banwart 1984). Fischer and Phillips (2006) recently demonstrated the efficacy of the essential oil of bergamot in significantly reducing populations of *E. coli* O157 and *C. jejuni*. In this study the Gram-positive bacteria tested appeared to be more sensitive than the Gram-negative bacteria.

TriSodiumPhosphate

TSP (trisodium phosphate) is employed in the United States to reduce numbers of *Campylobacter* and other contaminants present on poultry carcasses. In this country, the treatment is generally carried out after refrigeration by plunging the carcasses in a bath of 10 % TSP at 50°C for 15 s (Slavik et al., 1994). This procedure decreases the mean level of contamination of the poultry by 1.2 to 1.5 logs. In France, Federighi et al. (1995) obtained a reduction of 1.3 logs in the mean level of contamination of chicken carcasses by thermotolerant *Campylobacter*, the treatment being performed after evisceration, before refrigeration.

Disinfectants

Campylobacter do not seem to display any particular resistance to the disinfectants commonly used in the food industry, although few works have been devoted to this subject. An *in vitro* study by Avrain et al. (2003) showed that treatment with benzalkonium chloride (1 %) or sodium hypochlorite (0.63 %) allowed easy elimination of several strains of *Campylobacter*.

Broccoli Extracts

Recently, two isothiocyanates extracted from broccoli showed interesting anti-*Campylobacter* activity, bactericidal rather than bacteriostatic. The collection of 24 strains tested failed to show a different behavior in strains of different origins (Dufour et al. 2012).

Conclusion

Its strong presence in the digestive tract of many animals and its ability to cause disease in humans explain that *Campylobacter jejuni* is a major zoonotic agent, recognized all over the world. The disease it causes, called campylobacteriosis digestive, is generally not considered very serious except for certain categories of people who are more fragile. By cons, some complications that follow a digestive campylobacteriosis, such as Guillain-Barré syndrome, are very serious. The control of *Campylobacter* requires actions at two levels:

- By developing strategies to control *Campylobacter* throughout the food production chain, in order to reduce the incidence of the disease among consumers.
- And, by developing new and effective medical treatments.

Research should continue to grow for the two levels but, it is necessary, according to the "One Health" concept, to increase the level of mutual understanding of the laboratories, often working in parallel. This is the price to pay for the control of *Campylobacter* and its consequences for humans.

References

Abeyta C, Deeter FG, Kaysner CA, Stott RF, Wekell MM (1993). *Campylobacter jejuni* in a Washington state selfish growing bed associated with illness. *J Food Protect*, 56(4) : 323-325.

Al-Sakkaf A (2012). Evaluation of food handling practice among New Zealanders and other developed countries as a main risk factor for campylobacteriosis rate. *Food Control*, 27: 330-337.

Alter T, Scherer K (2006). Stress response of *Campylobacter* spp. and its role in food processing. *J. Vet. Med.*, B 53 : 351-357.

Avrain L, Allain L, Vernozy-Rozand C, Kempf I (2003). Disinfectants susceptibility testing of avain and swine *Campylobacter* isolates by a filtration method. *Vet Microbiol*, 96(1): 35-40.

Baré J, Uyttendaele M, Habib I, Depraetere O, Houf K, De Zutter L (2013). Variation in *Campylobacter* distribution on different sites of broiler carcasses. *Food Control*, 32: 279-282.

Bashor MP, Curtis PA, Keener KM, Sheldon BW, Kathariou S, Osborne JA (2004). Effects of carcass washers on *Campylobacter* contamination in large broiler processing plants. *Poultry Sci,* 83 : 1232-1239.

Bièche C, Ritz M, Tresse O, Federighi M, de Lamballerie M (2009). Impacts of treatment parameters on the inactivation of *Campylobacter jejuni* by high pressure: a statistical study of main effects and interactions. *Lett Appl Microbiol,* 48: 198-202.

Bhaduri S, Cottrell B (2004). Survival of cold-stressed *Campylobacter jejuni* on ground chicken and chicken skin during frozen storage. *Appl. Environ. Microbiol.,* 70 : 7103-7109.

Black RE, Levine MM, Clements ML, Hughes TP, Blaser MJ (1988). Experimental *Campylobacter jejuni* infections in humans. *J Infect Dis,* 157 : 472-479.

Butler RC, Lund V, Carlson DA (1987). Susceptibility of *Campylobacter jejuni* and *Yersinia enterocolitica* to UV Radiation. *Appl Environ Microbiol*, 53(2) : 375-378.

Chai LC, Robin T, Ragavan UM, Gunsalam JW, Abubakar F, Ghazali FM, Radu S, Kumar MP 2007. Thermophilic *Campylobacter* spp. in salad vegetables in Malaysia. *Int J Food Microbiol*, 117(1) : 106-111.

Choi HK, Marth EH, Vasadava PC (1993). Use of microwave to inactivate *Yersinia enterocolitica* and *Campylobacter jejuni* in milk. *Milchwissenschaft*, 48 : 134-136.

Deibel KE, Banwart GJ (1984). Effect of spices on *C. jejuni* at three temperatures. *J Food Safety*, 6(4) : 241-251.

Doorduyn Y, Van Den Bradhof WE, Van Duynhoven YT, Breukink BJ, Wagenaar JA, Van Pelt W (2010). Risk factors for indigenous *Campylobacter jejuni* and *Campylobacter coli* infections in The Netherlands: a case-control study. *Epidemiol Infect,* 138(10): 1391-1404.

Dufour V, Alazzam B, Ermel G, Thepaut M, Rossero A, Tresse O, Baysse C (2012). Antimicrobial activities of isothiocyanates against *Campylobacter jejuni* isolates. *Front Cell Infect Microbiol*, 2 : 53-60.

Dykes GA, Moorhead SM, (2001). Survival of *Campylobacter jejuni* on vacuum or carbon dioxide packaged primal beef cuts stored à -1.5°C. *Food Control*, 12 : 553-557.

Elmnasser N, Guillou S, Leroi F, Orange N, Bakhrouf A, Federighi M (2007). Pulsed light system as a novel food decontamination technology: a review. *Can J Microbiol*, 53: 813-821.

EFSA (2012) *Rapport annuel.* Autorité européenne de sécurité des aliments, Parme (consultable en ligne http://www.efsa.europa.eu/fr/corporate/doc /ar12fr.pdf).

EFSA (2013) *Annual report.* European food safety authority, Parme (consultable en ligne http://www.efsa.europa.eu/fr/corporate/doc/ar13. pdf).

Evans M, Ribeiro CD, Salmon RL (2003). Hazards of healthy living: bottled water and salad vegetables as risk factors for *Campylobacter* infection. *Emerg Infect Dis,* 9 : 1219-1225.

Federighi M, Cappelier JM, Rossero A, Coppen P, Denis JC (1995). Evaluation de l'effet d'un traitement de décontamination de carcasses de poulets, vis-à-vis des *Campylobacter* thermotolérants. *Sci Alim*, 15 : 393-401.

Federighi M, Tholozan JL, Cappelier JM, Tissier JP, Jouve JL (1998). Evidence of non coccoid viable but non culturable *Campylobacter jejuni* cells in microcosm water by direct viable count, CTC-DAPI double staining and scanning electron microscopy. *Food Microbiol*, 15(5) : 539-550.

Federighi M (1999a) *Campylobacter et hygiène des aliments*. Polytechnica, Paris.

Federighi M, Magras C, Pilet MF, (2005). *Campylobacter. In* Federighi M. (ed.) *Bactériologie alimentaire : Compendium d'hygiène des aliments*. Economica, Paris, 145-172.

Federighi M, Magras C, Pilet MF, Woodward DL, Johnson W, Jugiau F, Jouve JL (1999b). Incidence of thermotolerant *Campylobacter* in foods assessed by NF-ISO 10272: results of a two year study. *Food Microbiol*, 16(2) : 195-204.

Federighi M, Pilet MF, Woodward DL, Cappelier JM, Minet J, Johnson WM, Jouve JL (1997). Isolation of *Campylobacter jejuni* from retail trade oysters (*Crassostrea gigas*). *Microbiol Alim Nutr*, 15 : 41-45.

Federighi M, (2007). *Campylobacter jejuni* and food safety: microaerophilic and thermotolerant pathogen. *In :* Berger MC (ed.*) New developments in food microbiology research*. Nova Sciences Publishers, New York, 3-13.

Fisher K, Phillips C (2006). The effect of lemon, orange and bergamot essential oils and their components on the survival of *Campylobacter jejuni*, *Escherichia coli* O157, *Listeria monocytogenes*, *Bacillus cereus* and *Staphylococcus aureus in vitro* and in food systems. *J Appl Microbiol*, 101 : 1232-1240.

Friedman C, Nieman J, Wegener H, Tauxe R (2000). Epidemiology of *Campylobacter jejuni* infections in the United States and other industrialised nations. *In* : Nachamkin I, Blaser MJ. *Campylobacter*. ASM Press, Washington, 121-138.

Gallay A, De Valk H, Cournot M, Ladeuil B, Hemery C, Castor C, Bon F, Mégraud F, Le Cann P, Desenclos JC (2006). A large multi-pathogen waterborne community outbreak linked to faecal contamination of a groundwater system, France. *Clin Microbiol Infect*, 12(6) : 561-570.

Guerry P (2007). *Campylobacter* flagella: not just for motility. *Trends Microbiol*, 15: 456-461.

Guillou, S, Leguerinel I, Garrec N, Renard MA, Cappelier JM, Federighi M (2008). Survival of *Campylobacter jejuni* in mineral bottled water according to difference in mineral content: application of the Weibull model. *Water Research*, 42(8-9) : 2213-9.

Haughton PN, Gomez-Grau E, Lyng J, Cronin D, Fanning S, Whyte P (2012). Susceptibility of *Campylobacter* to high intensity near ultraviolet/visible 395±5 nm light and its effectiveness for the decontamination of raw chicken and contact surfaces. *Int J Food Microbiol*, 159 : 267-273.

Jacob-Reitsma W, Lyhs U, Wagenaar J (2008). *Campylobacter* in the food supply. *In* : Nachamkin I, Szymanski CM, Blaser MJ. *Campylobacter (third edition).* ASM Press, Washington, 627-644.

Juven BJ, Kanner J, Weisslowicz H, Harel S (1988). Effect of ascorbic and isoascorbic acids on survival of *Campylobacter jejuni* in poultry meat. *J Food Prot*, 51 : 436-437.

Kusumaningrum HD, Riboldi G, Hazeleger WC.,Beumer RR (2003). Survival of foodborne pathogens on stainless steel surfaces and cross-contamination to foods. *Int J Food Microbiol,* 85 : 227-236.

Konkel M, Joens L, Mixter P (2000). Molecular characterization of *Campylobacter jejuni* virulence determinants. *In* : Nachamkin I and Blaser MJ. *Campylobacter.* ASM Press, Washington, 217-240.

Lewis SJ, Velasquez A, Cuppet SL, Mckee, SR (2002). Effect of electron beam irradiation on poultry meat safety and quality. *Poult Sci*, 81 : 896-903.

Martinez-Rodriguez A, Mackey BM (2005). Factors affecting the pressure resistance of some *Campylobacter* species. *Lett Appl Microbiol*, 41 : 321-326.

Messaoudi S, Manaï M, Federighi M, Dousset X (2013). *Campylobacter* dans la filière poulet : étude bibliographique des stratégies de maîtrise au stade de l'élevage. *Rev Méd Vét*, 164(2) : 90-99.

Messaoudi S, Kergourlay G, Dalgallarondo M, Choiset Y, Ferchichi M, Prévost H, Pilet MF, Chobert JM, Manai M, Dousset X (2012). Purification and characterization of a new bacteriocin active against *Campylobacter* produced by *Lactobacillus salivarius* SMXD51. *Food Microbiol*, 32(1) : 129-134.

Müller A, Leon-Kempis M, Dodson E, Wilson K, Wilkinson A, Kelly D (2007). A Bacterial virulence factor with a dual role as an adhesin and a solute-binding protein: the crystal structure at 1.5 A resolution of the PEB1a protein from the food-borne human pathogen *Campylobacter jejuni. J Mol Biol*, 372 : 160-171.

Murdoch LE, Maclean M, Macgregor SJ, Anderson JG (2010). Inactivation of *Campylobacter jejuni* by exposure to high-intensity 405-nm visible light. *Foodborne Pathog Dis*, 7: 1211-1216.

Park CE, Sanders GW (1992). Occurrence of thermotolerant *campylobacters* in fresh vegetables *Can J Microbiol*, 38: 313-316

Remize F, Montagné E, Lucan A, Aviat F, Federighi M (2013). Prévalence de *Campylobacter* sur les magrets de canard et influence de la transformation par séchage. *VPC,* janvier 2013, 1-7.

Schoeni JL, Doyle MP (1992). Reduction of *Campylobacter jejuni*colonization of chicks by caecum-colonizing bacteria producing anti-*C.jejuni*metabolites. *Appl Environ Microbiol*, 58(2) : 664-670

Silva J, Leite D, Fernandes M, Mena C, Gibbs PA, Teixeira P (2011). *Campylobacter* spp. as a foodborne pathogen: a review. *Front Microbiol*, 2(200) : 1-12.

Slavik FM, Kim JW, Pharr MD, Raben DP, Tsai S, Lobs CM, (1994) Effect of triSodium Phosphate on *Campylobacter* attached to post-chilled chicken carcasses. *J. Food Prot.*, 57, 324-326.

Solomon EB, Hoover DG (2004). Inactivation of *Campylobacter jejuni* by high hydrostatic pressure. *Lett Appl Microbiol*, 38 : 505-509.

Stern NJ, Svetoch EA, Eruslanov BV, Perelygin VV, Mitsevich EV, Mitsevich IP, Pokhilenko VD, Levchuk VP, Svetoch OE, Seal BS (2006). Isolation of a *Lactobacillus salivarius* strain and purification of its bacteriocin, which is inhibitory to *Campylobacter jejuni* in the chicken gastrointestinal system. *Antimicrob Agents Chemother*, 50 : 3111-3116.

Vellinga A, Van Loock F (2002). The dioxin crisis as experiment to determine poultry-related campylobacter enteritis. *Emerg Infect Dis,* 8 : 19-22.

Young K, Davis L, DiRita V (2007). *Campylobacter jejuni*: molecular biology and pathogenesis. *Nat Rev Microbiol*, 5 : 665-679.

In: Campylobacter Infections
Editor: Brittany A. Bertucci

ISBN: 978-1-63463-858-6

Chapter 3

Campylobacteriosis Associated with Mass Catering: A Survey on the European Union Cases

Andrea Osimani[1,*] ***and Francesca Clementi***[1]
[1]Dipartimento di Scienze Agrarie, Alimentari ed Ambientali, Università Politecnica delle Marche, Ancona, Italy

Abstract

The genus *Campylobacter* comprises Gram-negative spiral-shaped bacteria, which can cause a foodborne illness in humans called campylobacteriosis; the infection generally occurs through the consumption of undercooked chicken or ready-to-eat meals that have been in contact with contamined raw chicken. The occurrence of pathogens in foods may be caused by cross-contamination, mainly due to insufficient hygiene of the staff and the environment, and/or by improper conditions enabling survival and growth of microorganisms, like inadequate cooking or temperature abuse.

In Europe, the general principles and requisites of food safety legislation have been established by Regulation (EC) 178/2002, followed by Regulation (EC) 852/2004 on the hygiene of foodstuffs. One of the basic obligations foreseen by Regulation (EC) 852/2004 is that food businesses operators have to implement permanent procedures based on

* Tel.: +39-071-2204959, Fax: +39-071-2204988, E-mail: a.osimani@univpm.it.

Hazard Analysis and Critical Control Point (HACCP) principles in order to ensure the safety of products.

In recent years, public catering has taken on an increasingly important role in the lives of working people, and food safety linked to the consumption of out-of-home meals has become a critical issue; in particular, the increase in the cases of campylobacteriosis highlights the need for continuous monitoring and control of the presence of *Campylobacter* spp. in the food chain.

The European Food Safety Authority (EFSA) estimates that the cost of the episodes of campylobacteriosis for the health system, in terms of lost productivity in the European Union, is around € 2.4 billion a year. Recent microbiological studies conducted in the United Kingdom, Ireland, Spain and Denmark showed that cases of *Campylobacter* infection (well recognised or not) depended largely upon an incorrect application of good manufacturing procedures, hygiene related to the handling of raw materials (mainly poulty meat) and cooking. This last procedure was recognised as one of the main critical points. To date, the Commission Decision (EC) 516/2007 regulates the tolerance to the presence of thermotolerant species of *Campylobacter* on slaughtered carcasses, but it does not specify tolerances for foods ready for consumption, as already provided for other pathogens such as *Salmonella* spp. and *Listeria monocytogenes*. Though current European legislation on zoonoses requires prompt notification of episodes of human infectious diseases to the National Health System, a lack of official data occurs in several European Countries because of the absence of harmonized procedures for monitoring and recording the cases of campylobacteriosis.

Introduction

The genus *Campylobacter* includes Gram-negative spiral-shaped bacteria (0.2-0.9 µm x 0.2-0.5 µm), which can grow at temperatures between 37°C and 45°C, with an optimum at 42°C; moreover, the growth is quite slow or even absent between 21°C and 30°C. Most of *Campylobacter* species associated with human diseases require 3-5% oxygen and 2-10% carbon dioxide for growth (Forsythe, 2010). Since *Campylobacter* spp. are fragile microorganisms, they are susceptible to heat treatments such as cooking and/or pasteurization and freezing, use of brine and acids, and to the use of disinfectants.

Within the genus *Campylobacter*, thermotolerant species including *Campylobacter jejuni, Campylobacter coli, Campylobacter lari* and *Campylobacter upsaliensis* are often associated with gastrointestinal illness in humans. The illness is called campylobacteriosis, and the major symptoms include flu-like illness, abdominal pain, fever and diarrhoea (watery and often bloody in children) (Forsythe, 2010). The infection dose comprises between 500 and 1,000 cells, and the incubation period varies from 2 to 10 days with an average time of 4 days. Since the infection is self-limiting, treatment mainly consists in electrolyte replacement and rehydration; in some invasive cases, antimicrobial treatment (erythromycin, tetracycline, quinolones) can be recommended (WHO, 2011). Infection has been associated with complications such as joint inflammation (5–10% of cases) and, on rare occasions, Guillain–Barré syndrome, a temporary but severe paralysis that may result in death (ECDC, 2013).

Usually, the species belonging to the genus *Campylobacter* are not environmental microorganisms but are associated with warm-blooded animals. In fact, a wide range of meat animals such as swine, cattle and birds contain *C. jejuni* in their oral cavities, intestinal and urogenital tracts (Altekruse 1999). In more detail, several investigations have reported that *C. jejuni* was found in chicken and swine intestinal contents and carcasses, swine and sheep feces, and eviscerated chicken and turkey (Jay et al., 2005). Beside livestock, thermotolerant *Campylobacter* spp. can also contaminate water and raw milk. Tough poultry is considered the most important potential source of infections which, via cross-contamination, represents a major risk for consumer health, especially when inadequate preparation and manipulation of contaminated raw meat are carried out (Forsythe, 2010). In the year 2014, the European Food Safety Authority (EFSA) and the European Centre for Disease Prevention and Control (ECDC) reported that 23.6 % of the samples (single or batch) of fresh broiler meat were found to be positive for *Campylobacter* in the reporting Member States (MSs), which was less than in 2011, when 31.3 % of the samples were positive. However, the list of MSs involved in 2011 and 2012 reports were not exactly the same; therefore, the whole set of data is not comparable. In addition, for the MSs, included in both years' reports, there were discrepancies regarding the prevalence of *Campylobacter* in the reported proportions of positive samples compared with 2011.

Globally, the high number of case-studies analysed by EFSA and ECDC highlighted that in 2012, the notification rate and the number of confirmed cases of campylobacteriosis in humans in the European Union (EU) showed a drop in relation to those recorded in 2011. Notwithstanding, human campylobacteriosis still remains the most frequently reported zoonosis with 214,268 confirmed cases (EFSA and ECDC, 2014). In fact, the magnitude of *Campylobacter* spp. infections reported in the EU followed a significant increasing trend in 2008-2012, (with a clear seasonal trend); in addition, the percentage of *Campylobacter*-positive food and animal samples in 2012 remained at levels similar to those in previous years, with a constant high occurrence of *Campylobacter* spp. in broiler meat (EFSA, and ECDC, 2014). Fortunately, given the high number of campylobacteriosis cases, the percentage of fatalities reported can be considered to be quite low (0.03 %) (EFSA and ECDC, 2014).

Mass Catering Concerns and the European Food Safety Approach

In recent years, the trend towards eating in restaurants, fast-food outlets and canteens has been growing, and the number of fast food restaurants has notably increased. Although much has been done to improve food safety and reduce risks for consumer health within acceptable limits, achieving zero risk level cannot be considered realistically feasible, even in the most advanced societies (Cenci Goga and Clementi, 2002).

Within the long way towards an increasingly high level of food safety, the introduction of a preventive approach (forward control), focussed on the process (processing, storage, distribution) can be considered an important milestone. This novel approach, joined to the traditional products inspection (backward control) was introduced in the EU with the Directive (EC) 93/43, which made the application of the Hazard Analysis and Critical Control Point (HACCP) system mandatory across the food industry, with the exception of primary production. The implementation of the HACCP system is based on five preliminary steps: (i) formation of the HACCP team; (ii) product description; (iii) identification of the intended use; (iv) flow chart construction; (v) on-site confirmation of flow charts; and seven principles: (i) hazard identification; (ii) determination of critical control points (CCP); (iii) identification of critical limits; (iv) set-up of monitoring procedures; (v) organization of corrective action; (vi) set-up of procedures to verify that the HACCP system was working as intended; and (vii) organization of recordkeeping procedures. Before implementing the HACCP plan, basic good hygiene conditions and practices (known as prerequisites) must be defined as well. Prerequisites (when appropriate) include: food environment cleaning and sanitation (Osimani et al., 2014), maintenance, hygiene and training of the staff, pest control, plant and equipment, premises and structure, ancillary services (water, ice, steam, compressed air, ventilation, etc.), storage, transport and distribution, waste management, zoning (physical separation of activities to prevent potential food contamination). Once all the appropriate prerequisites are respected and the HACCP plan is implemented, this preventive approach could control all the steps of the production process that are critical for ensuring the preparation of safe food (Panisello et al., 2000). In order to fully accomplish this aim, food businesses are recommended to use appropriate standards for each sector (e.g., processing, catering, retail).

Though the principles set by Directive (EC) 93/43 still inspires the European legislation on food safety today, further changes have been introduced by the EU in the wake of several food scandals in order to reinforce the regulatory control on food hygiene issues and to re-gain the compromised trust of citizens. To this aim, in January 2002, the framework Regulation (EC) 178/2002 was adopted, followed by the publication of four acts in 2004 which formed the so-called "Food Hygiene Package": Regulation (EC) 852/2004 on the hygiene of foodstuffs which replaced Directive (EC) 93/43; Regulation (EC) 853/2004 laying down specific hygiene rules for food of animal origin, Regulation (EC) 854/2004 laying down specific rules for the organization of official controls on products of animal origin intended for human consumption, and Regulation (EC) 882/2004 on official controls performed to ensure the verification of compliance with feed and food law, animal health and animal welfare rules. Subsequently, Regulation (EC) 2073/2005, as amended by Regulation (EC) 1441/2007 concerning the microbiological criteria for food safety and process hygiene, established, for the first time, a long list of critical limits for pathogenic foodborne bacteria including their toxins and metabolites. To date, the Decision (EC) 516/2007 regulates tolerance to the presence of thermotolerant species of *Campylobacter* on slaughtered carcasses but does not specify the limits for foods, as established in Regulation (EC) 2073/2005 for other pathogens such as *Salmonella* spp. and *Listeria monocytogenes* (Petruzzeli et al., 2010).

The application of the HACCP system is particularly complex in the catering sector because of some peculiarities that it presents, such as the variety of raw materials and ingredients processed, the numerous flow-charts applied, and the large number of (different) meals served daily (Osimani et al., 2013a, 2013b; Petruzzelli et al., 2014a). For these reasons, catering is still responsible for a significant proportion of infections and intoxications of food origin (Maruzumi et al., 2005; Black et al., 2006; Brila et al., 2006; Medus et al., 2006; Moffatt et al., 2006). Despite the mandatory application of the HACCP system, many risk factors are still not adequately controlled, such as:

(i) raw materials contaminated with pathogens, (ii) inadequate hygiene of the environment and staff, (iii) inadequate conditions of cooking and storage of foods (Osimani et al., 2011).

In order to protect consumers from the risk related to the presence of *Campylobacter* spp. in foods, the EU adopted an integrated approach to food safety that involves the entire supply chain, from farm to table. This approach, supported by timely and effective communication activities on the risks, includes risk assessment and risk management carried out by the MSs, the European Commission and Parliament, the EFSA and the ECDC. In order to gain insight into the frequency of *Campylobacter* contamination in raw meat and in foods in the year 2008, an EU-wide baseline survey on *Campylobacter* in broiler batches and on broiler carcasses was carried out (EFSA, 2010); in the year 2011, a Scientific Opinion on *Campylobacter* in broiler meat production was drawn up by the EFSA Panel on Biological Hazards (EFSA, 2011). Recently, the EFSA and the ECDC provided overviews on EU reports on trends and sources of zoonoses, zoonotic agents and food-borne outbreaks, including campylobacteriosis frequencies in humans and *Campylobacter* presence in foods and animals (EFSA and ECDC 2013, 2014). Currently, as concerns foods, the presence of *Campylobacter* spp. is notifiable in the following EU MSs: Austria, Belgium, the Czech Republic, Estonia (only *C. jejuni*), Germany, Iceland, Italy, Latvia, Norway, the Netherlands, Poland, Slovakia, Slovenia and Spain (EFSA and ECDC, 2014).

Case Reports

The current economic and technical developments along with new production systems have made the food chain longer and more complex, thus increasing the possibilites for contamination ond/or microbial surviving and growth during food processing. Negligences in the application of the good manufacturing practices (GMP) by the personnel operating at catering facilities and, in particular, undercooking of foods of animal origin are important factors in the outbreaks of food-borne illnesses, as confirmed by recent studies, described below, which emphasize the importance of proper management of food handling, also in relation to the risk associated with the presence of *Campylobacter*.

In 2006, Whyte et al. carried out a study for the assessment of cooking conditions required for the inactivation of naturally present *Campylobacter* cells in chicken livers. The analysis carried out on chicken liver samples showed a high level of contamination with the presence of *Campylobacter* spp. in 90% of the samples. The same study highlighted the contribution of the preparation of chicken liver recipes in the eventual survival of *Campylobacter*; in particular, it emerged that many of the recipes require that the liver, after cooking, remain pink in the middle, thus allowing microbial survival. Whyte *et al.* determined that, in order to be considered free from *Campylobacter*, chicken liver should reach a temperature of 70 °C at the core of the product for at least 2-5 minutes. Therefore, although a pink-in-the-middle liver could be particularly appreciated by the consumer, it does not guarantee safety of the product.

A study published by Mazick et al. (2006) has identified for the first time in Denmark a major outbreak of *Campylobacter* infection associated with contaminated chicken from France, processed in an industrial kitchen serving the employees of three companies. The link between the employees' foodborne illness and food served at the canteens was established by administering questionnaires to the employees. From the analysis of the data it seemed plausible that the transmission of the infection was related to cross-contamination mainly due to improper handling practices of the processed food in the kitchen under investigation. This confirmed the importance of stringent preventive measures to prevent cross-contamination during handling of poultry meats. The data reported in the study also suggested that for each case of recorded campylobacteriosis, 20 undiagnosed cases might actually occur.

Analogously, a brief report carried out by Calciati et al. (2012) found that deficient kitchen facilities associated with poor hygiene of food preparation practices appeared to be the key issues for cross-contamination of *Campylobacter* from raw chicken to cooked food in 75 primary school in Barcelona (Spain) which served roast chicken and Russian salad.

Inadequate cooking of chicken liver was reported as a significant risk factor in a paper published by O'Leary et al. (2009); the study started as a consequence of an outbreak of campylobacteriosis affecting 48 people who had eaten lunch at a restaurant in Forth Valley (Scotland, UK). The presence of *Campylobacter* in chicken liver was presumably imputable to a change in the preparation procedure of the liver which was neither followed by a reassessment of the hazards nor by the implementation of the required verifications to guarantee the safety of the end product. The research found the first documented continuous outbreak source of *Campylobacter* in Scotland.

In the year 2010, Little et al. published a short report in which they highlighted the contribution of food catering services in the transmission of

Campylobacter in the UK. In particular, the research showed that 64% of cases of infection were linked to restaurants and hotels. The study by Little *et al.* also confirmed that poultry (meat and liver pâté) is the main vehicle of infection followed by drinking water and milk. Little et al. also identified the major causes of the presence of the infective agent which, similar to that discovered by O'Leary et al. (2009), were modifications of the cooking procedures that favoured the survival of *Campylobacte*r, while inadequate hygiene measures were found to be responsible for promoting cross-contaminations between raw and processed foods. Little and co-workers also highlighted the importance of implementation, monitoring and verification procedures for the handling of processed food in public catering facilities in accordance with the provisions of Regulation (EC) 852/2004.

Farmer and colleagues in 2012 published a study which was undertaken as a result of episodes of campylobacteriosis associated with the consumption of chicken liver served in a restaurant in the urban area of Liverpool (UK). Environmental surveys and interviews with kitchen staff highlighted that the improper food preparation procedures could allow cross-contamination of other food products, especially during the preparation of chicken livers. The same study also showed the need for a rapid notification of cases of infection in order to facilitate the collection of samples for microbiological analyses for prompt investigation on potential outbreaks.

A study carried out by Abid et al. (2013) reported the data about a campylobacteiosis outbreak that occurred in 2011 in the United Kingdom, which involved two groups of people (consisting of 3 and 29 persons, respectively) who had had lunch in a college restaurant. In order to establish the origin of the infection, health officers were involved; they first reviewed the diets consumed by the sick persons, and the cause of the disease was attributed to the consumption of duck liver pâté. The Authors concluded that the outbreak occurred because of the inadequacy of the procedures for the preparation of liver pâté. Furthermore, it was highlighted that the raw liver was cooked improperly without ensuring that the core of the product had reached 70 °C for at least 2-5 minutes, as already recommended by Whyte et al. (2006).

A recent study by Petruzzelli et al. (2014b) investigated the frequency of thermotolerant *Campylobacter* in raw meat samples collected in Italy from 2006 to 2012 at different catering facilities (schools, hospitals and military barracks), in order to obtain data for subsequent use in risk-assessment. Statistical analysis of the data showed a significantly higher frequency of the pathogen in poultry meat (22.1%) than in red meat (5.5%). Petruzzelli et al.

also highlighted an evident increase in positive samples in 2011 within the poultry meat analysed.

The study carried out by Petruzzelli et al., showed how the potential risk of cross-contamination can be real and reiterated the need to pay attention to the handling of raw materials (poultry and red meats) in the catering food production environment. Indeed, the presence of *Campylobacter* was not negligible, although, in this study, data on the actual microbial load of the microrganism were not produced. As a conclusion of their study, the Authors suggested that in order to arrive at an accurate representation of the level of contamination of thermotolerant *Campylobacter*, a national surveillance system should be set up.

As is evident from the analysis of the scientific literature, the cases of *Campylobacter* infection (well recognised or not) depend largely upon an incorrect application of GMP related to the handling of raw materials (especially poultry meat) and cooking, the latter aspect is recognised as one of the main critical points. Indeed, it is worth noticing that a GMP is that part of quality assurance which ensures that products are consistently produced and controlled to the quality standards appropriate to their intended use and as required by the marketing authorization; a GMP is one of the main prerequisites that can prevent risks related to food processing. Therefore, greater attention should be paid towards the validation of the procedures that have been found to be critical in combination with a more careful training of the personnel which processes foods. Currently, it is not possible to guarantee that raw materials are free from pathogens. Therefore, it is essential to implement appropriate preventive and control measures involving the whole food production chain in order to prevent cross-contamination and survival/multiplication of *Campylobacter*. The preventive measures which can be used as concerns the raw material may be related to appropriate packaging (Donnison and Ross, 2004), whereas, with regard to the end product (ready-to-eat), it is necessary to ensure a clear separation from raw materials and an accurate control of cooking (i.e., 70 °C for at least 2-5 minutes for chicken liver) and maintenance temperatures until meal distribution (Donnison and Ross, 2004). The effectiveness of the cooking process depends on several factors, such as: the microbiological quality of raw meats, the amount of meat to be cooked, the size of the piece(s), the cooking method (frying, roasting, boiling, etc.), the type of equipment used for cooking (oven, crock pot, stew pot, grill, etc.), the presence of additional ingredients (potatoes, stuffing, raw parsley, sauces, spices, etc.). In addition, efficient protection from post-cooking contaminations, rapid cooling down (by blast-chillers) and controlled cold storage are all factors of primary importance for guaranteeing safety of the cooked meat preparations (Daelman et al., 2013; Gibbons et al., 2006; Juneja et al., 2001; Mataragas et al., 2008).

As an example of the attention that the EU MSs are giving to the problem of campylobacteriosis, the information campaign lounched by the UK Food Standard Agency (FSA) in 2014 can be mentioned. This initiative was aimed at communicating the risks related to the spread of *Campylobacter* in the food preparation environment during the washing of raw chicken meat before cooking.

The Scientific Report of the EFSA and the ECDC on Trends and Sources of Zoonoses, Zoonotic Agents and Food-borne Outbreaks in 2012 reported that within the EU, 19 MSs reported a total of 501 food-borne campylobacteriosis outbreaks, less than those (596) recorded in 2011 (9.3 and 10.6 % of the total reported food-borne outbreaks in the EU, respectively). The overall reporting rate in the EU was 0.10 per 100,000 population, similar to that reported in 2011 (0.12) and in 2010 (0.10). Furthermore, Austria, Germany and Slovakia reported the majority of outbreaks (78.2 %). In addition, Norway and Switzerland reported two outbreaks each. Only 25 (5.0 %) of the campylobacteriosis outbreaks were classified as strong-evidence outbreaks. Moreover, Switzerland reported two strong-evidence outbreaks, one of which involved a fatal case (EFSA and ECDC, 2014).

The EFSA and the ECDC reports stated that 19 out of the 25 strong-evidence *Campylobacter* outbreaks in Europe were classified as general outbreaks, the remaining four as household outbreaks, and just two were classified as unknown. In 2012, broiler meat was most frequently identified as food vehicle (44.0 % of outbreaks). The percentage of strong-evidence outbreaks implicating broiler meat was quite similar to that in 2011 (45.9 %) (EFSA and ECDC, 2014).

Six out of the 7 outbreaks reported by the United Kingdom were associated with broiler meat, while of the 5 outbreaks reported by France, 2 were associated with broiler meat and the other 3 with meats of other animals (bovine, or mixed red and turkey meat). The 5 outbreaks reported by Germany were associated with meat preparations such as minced pig meat (1 outbreak), *carpaccio* from raw duck meat (1 outbreak), or with raw milk (3 outbreaks).

Mass catering meals (at restaurant, café, pub, bar, hotel, catering service) were identified in 10 out of 21 outbreaks, being the most frequently origin reported, followed by household/domestic meals (kitchen) for 6 outbreaks. Many contributory factors, either alone or in combination, were reported in 14 outbreaks. The most common factor was inadequate heat treatment (5 outbreaks), followed by unprocessed contaminated ingredient (4 outbreaks). Two outbreaks were reported by Switzerland: both were general outbreaks associated with broiler meat. The origin of the outbreaks were meals served at a residential institution and at a mass catering facility, whereas the contributory factors were storage time/temperature abuse and cross-contamination, respectively (EFSA and ECDC, 2014).

Conclusion

Microbiological hazards and related issues continue to be major challenges to the safety of the meat and meat products. It is important to note that the management of risks along the meat chain must be based on an integrated effort that applies to all the sectors involved, including primary production, processing (and handling), packaging and distribution (Sofos, 2008).

As regards the risk of *Campylobacter* in 2002, the Food Safety Authority of Ireland (FSAI) reported some data that appeared in the Opinion of the Scientific Committee on Veterinary Measures relating to Public Health Zoonosis Food of the European Commission. This report stated that the main risk factors associated with sporadic campylobacteriosis are: i) improper handling of raw poultry; ii) undercooked poultry meat and/or cooked on the grill, poultry liver, pork or sausages; iii) contact with puppies or cats (diarrhea); iv) non-potable water, contaminated raw milk or unpasteurized dairy products; v) travel abroad.

To ensure an effective control on direct and indirect contamination that usually comes from carcasses of slaughtered animals, it is extremely important to implement hygiene management procedures during the food production process, which could minimize the risk of cross-contamination between raw materials, environment, and food ready for consumption. Within this context it is therefore necessary a correct risk assessment related to the presence of specific pathogens in foods with both epidemiological and microbiological approaches (Nørrung and Buncic, 2008).

As concerns *Campylobacter* risk management, in 2002, the FSAI issued some guidelines specifically conceived for food handlers in restaurants, cafés, canteens, supermarkets and corner shops, since they have to deal with the remaining contamination coming from the earlier parts of the food chain and prevent contaminated food from entering the food chain; the control measures listed by the FSAI includes: (i) prevention of contamination from contaminated water, unhygienic premises, unhygienic food handler/food handling practices; (ii) prevention of cross-contamination between raw materials and ready-to-eat foods; (iii) appropriate storage and cooling to prevent bacterial multiplication; (iv) proper cooking or other treatments to kill microbial cells (FSAI, 2002; WHO, 2011). More recently, the EFSA and the ECDC confirmed that cross-contaminations between raw (poultry) meat and ready-to-eat meals during food preparation are important transmission routes of *Campylobacter*, though raw milk and contaminated drinking water have been implicated in both small and large outbreaks (EFSA and ECDC, 2014).

As concerns the EFSA's and ECDC's (2014) recent reports, it is worth noticing that, at the moment, the results, in terms of the presence of *Campylobacter* in foods obtained from different EU Countries, are not directly comparable owing to between-country variation in the sampling and testing methods used. It is also necessary to consider that the proportion of positive samples observed throughout the MSs could have been influenced by the sampling season since it is known that in many Countries *Campylobacter* infections are more prevalent during the summer than during the winter (EFSA and ECDC, 2014).

Although many advances have been made, presently, a lack of harmonized epidemiological data regarding food contamination in terms of load, frequency, and animal species makes the unique identification of the critical points of contamination and the extent of the hazard across the food chain uncertain (Laroche and Magras, 2013). As pointed out by Gölz et al. (2014), a multidisciplinary approach oriented to significantly reduce the burden of campylobacteriosis is strongly required; the strategy should include the main stakeholders such as: veterinary authorities, medical experts, scientists, policy makers, public health authorities, and the food industry.

References

Abid, M., Wimalarathna, H., Mills, J., Saldana, L., Pang, W., Richardson, J. F., Maiden, M. C., McCarthy, N. D. 2013. Duck liver-associated outbreak of campylobacteriosis among humans, United Kingdom, 2011. *Emerg. Infect. Dis.*, 19, 1310-1313.

Altekruse, S. F., Stern, N. J., Fields, P. I., Swerdlow, D. L., 1999. *Campylobacter jejuni*—An Emerging Foodborne Pathogen. *Emerg. Infec. Dis.*, 5, 28-35.

Analysis of the baseline survey on the prevalence of Campylobacter in broiler batches and of Campylobacter and Salmonella on broiler carcasses in the EU, 2008, Part A: Campylobacter and Salmonella prevalence estimates. *EFSA Journal*, 2010; 8(03):1503). [99 pp.]. doi:10.2903/j.efsa.2010.1503. Available online: www.efsa.europa.eu.

Black, A. P., Kirk, M. D., Millard, G., 2006. *Campylobacter* outbreak due to chicken consumption at an Australian Capital Territory restaurant. Commun. *Dis. Intell. Q. Rep.*, 30, 373–377.

Brila, A., Innuse, M., Perevoscikovs, J., Lucenko, I., 2006. An outbreak of *Salmonella enteritidis* infections linked to a restaurant in Riga, August 2006. *EuroSurveill*, 11:E061026.2.

Calciati, E., Lafuente, S., De Simó, M., Balfagon, P., Bartolomé, R., Caylà, J., 2012. A *Campylobacter* outbreak in a Barcelona school. *Enferm. Infecci. Microbiol. Clín.*, 30, 243–245.

Cenci Goga, B. T., Clementi, F., 2002. Safety assurance of foods: Risk management depends on good science but it is not a scientific activity. *J. Agr. Environ. Ethic,* 15, 305-313.

Commission Decision (EC) 2007/516 of 19 July 2007 concerning a financial contribution from the Community towards a survey on the prevalence and antimicrobial resistance of *Campylobacter* spp. in broiler flocks and on the prevalence of *Campylobacter* spp. and *Salmonella* spp. in broiler carcasses to be carried out in the Member States. *Official Journal of the European Union.*

Council Directive 93/43/EEC of 14 June 1993 on the hygiene of foodstuffs.

Daelman, J., Jacxsens, L., Lahou, E., Devlieghere, F., Uyttendaele, M., 2013. Assessment of the microbial safety and quality of cooked chilled foods and their production process. *Int. J. Food Microbiol.*, 160, 193–200.

Donnison, A. M., Ross, C. M., 2014. Microbiological safety of meat, Thermotolerant *Campylobacter*, Encyclopedia of Meat Sciences (Second Edition), pp. 382-388.

EFSA, (European Food Safety Authority), ECDC (European Centre for Disease Prevention and Control), 2013. The European Union Summary Report on Trends and Sources of Zoonoses, Zoonotic Agents and Food-borne Outbreaks in 2011; *EFSA Journal*, 2013;11(4):3129, 250 pp. doi:10.2903/j.efsa.2013.3129.

EFSA (European Food Safety Authority) and ECDC (European Centre for Disease Prevention and Control), 2014. The European Union Summary Report on Trends and Sources of Zoonoses, Zoonotic Agents and Foodborne Outbreaks in 2012. *EFSA Journal*, 2014;12(2):3547, 312 pp. doi:10.2903/j.efsa.2014.3547.

EFSA Panel on Biological Hazards (BIOHAZ); Scientific Opinion on Campylobacter in broiler meat production: control options and performance objectives and/or targets at different stages of the food chain. *EFSA Journal,* 2011;9(4):2105. [141 pp.]. doi:10.2903/j.efsa.2011.2105. Available online: www.efsa.europa.eu/efsajournal.

European Centre for Disease Prevention and Control (ECDC). Surveillance of food- and waterborne diseases in the EU/EEA – 2006–2009. Stockholm: ECDC; 2013.

Farmer, S., Keenan, A., Vivancos, R., 2012. Food-borne *Campylobacter* outbreak in Liverpool associated with cross-contamination from chicken liver parfait: Implications for investigation of similar outbreaks. *Public Health,* 126, 657-659.

Food Safety Authority of Ireland (FSAI). 2002. Control of *Campylobacter* species in the food chain. Food Safety Authority of Ireland, Abbey Court, Lower Abbey Street, Dublin 1.

Forsythe, S. J., 2010. The Microbiology of Safe Food, 2nd, Edition Wiley-Blackwell.

Gibbons, I., Adesiyun, A., Seepersadsingh, N., Rahaman, S., 2006. Investigation for possible source(s) of contamination of ready-to-eat meat products with Listeria spp. and other pathogens in a meat processing plant in Trinidad. *Food Microbiol.*, 23, 359–366.

Gölz, G., Rosner, B., Hofreuter, D., Josenhans, C., Kreienbrock, L., Löwenstein, A., Schielke, A., Stark, K., Suerbaum, S., Wieler, L. H., Alter, T., 2014. Relevance of *Campylobacter* to public health—The need for a One Health approach. *Int. J. Med. Microbiol.,* in press, http://dx.doi.org/10.1016/j.ijmm.2014.08.015.

Jay, J. M., Loessner, M. J, Golden, D. A., 2004. Modern Food Microbiology, 7th, Edition Springer.

Juneja, V. K., Marks, H., Huang, L., Thippareddi, H., 2001. Predictive model for growth of *Clostridium perfringens* during cooling of cooked uncured meat and poultry. *Food Microbiol.*, 28, 791-795.

Laroche, M., Magras, C., 2013. Gastrointestinal campylobacteriosis in industrialised countries: comparison of the disease situation with salmonellosis, and microbiological contamination assessment. *Rev. Sci. Tech.,* 32, 685-699.

Little, C. L., Gormley, F. J., Rawal, N., Richardson, J. F., 2010. A recipe for disaster: outbreaks of campylobacteriosis associated with poultry liver pâté in England and Wales. *Epidemiol. Infect.,* 138, 1691-1694.

Maruzumi, M., Morita, M., Matsuoka, Y., Uekawa, A., Nakamura, T., Fuji, K., 2005. Mass food poisoning caused by beef offal contaminated by *Escherichia coli* O157. Jpn. *J. Infect. Dis.,* 58, 397.

Mataragas, M., Skandamis, P. N., Drosinos, E. H., 2008. Risk profiles of pork and poultry meat and risk ratings of various pathogen/product combinations. *Int. J. Food Microbiol.,* 126, 1–12.

Mazick, A., Ethelberg, S., Møller Nielsen, E., Mølbak, K., Lisby, M., 2006. An outbreak of *Campylobacter jejuni* associated with consumption of chicken, Copenhagen, 2005. Eurosurveill. 11, 4-6.

Medus, C., Smith, K. E., Bender, J. B., Besser, J. M., Hedberg, C. W., 2006. *Salmonella* outbreaks in restaurants in Minnesota, 1995 through 2003: Evaluation of the role of infected food workers. *J. Food Protect.,* 69, 1870–1878.

Moffatt, C. R., Combs, B. G., Mwanri, L., Holland, R., Delroy, B., Cameron, S., Givney, R. C., 2006. An outbreak of *Salmonella typhimurium* phage type 64 gastroenteritis linked to catered luncheons in Adelaide, South Australia, June 2005. *Commun. Dis. Intell. Q. Rep.,* 30, 443–448.

Nørrung, B., Buncic, S., 2008. Microbial safety of meat in the European Union. *Meat Sci.,* 78, 14-24.

O'Leary, M. C., Harding, O., Fisher, L., Cowden, J., 2009. A continuous common source outbreak of campylobacteriosis associated with changes to the preparation of chicken liver pâté. *Epidemiol. Infect.,* 137, 383-388.

Osimani, A., Aquilanti, L., Clementi, F., 2014. Impiego del luminometro nella valutazione dello stato di pulizia delle superfici: il caso studio di una mensa universitaria. *Ind. Aliment-Italy,* 545, 12-18.

Osimani, A., Aquilanti, L., Clementi, F., 2013b. La verifica del sistema HACCP nella ristorazione collettiva: un caso studio. *Ind. Aliment-Italy,* 541, 18-25.

Osimani, A., Aquilanti, L., Tavoletti, S., Clementi F., 2013a. Evaluation of the HACCP system in a University Canteen: microbiological monitoring and internal auditing as verification tools. *Int. J. Environ. Res. Public Health,* 10, 1572-1585.

Osimani, A., Babini, V., Aquilanti, L., Tavoletti, S., Clementi, F., 2011. An eight-year report on the implementation of HACCP in a university canteen: impact on the microbiological quality of meals. *Int. J. Environ. Health Res.,* 21, 120–132.

Panisello, P. J., Rooney, R., Quantick, P. C., Stanwell-Smith, R., 2000. Application of foodborne disease outbreak data in the development and maintenance of HACCP systems. *Int. J. Food Microbiol.,* 59, 221–234.

Petruzzelli, A., Blasi, G., Masini, L., Calza, L., Duranti, A., Santarelli, S., Fisichella, S., Pezzetti, G., Aquilanti, L., Osimani, A., Tonucci, F., 2010. Occurrence of *Listeria monocytogenes* in Salami manufactured in the Marche region (Central Italy). *J. Vet. Med. Sci.,* 72, 499–502.

Petruzzelli, A., Foglini, M., Paolini, F., Framboas, M., Altissimi, M. S., Haouet, N. M., Mangili, P., Osimani, A., Clementi, F., Cenci, T., Tonucci, F., 2014a. Evaluation of the quality of foods for special diets produced in a school catering facility within a HACCP-based approach: a case study. *Int. J. Environ. Health Res.,* 24, 73-81.

Petruzzelli, A., Foglini, M., Vetrano, V., Paolini, F., Orazietti, N., Ambrosiani, B., Osimani, A., Clementi, F., Tavoletti, S., Tonucci, F., 2014b. The occurrence of thermotolerant *Campylobacter* spp. in raw meat intended for public catering. *Public Health*, 128, 388-390.

Regulation (EC) No. 178/2002 of the European Parliament and the Council of 28 January 2002 Laying down the General Principles and Requirements of Food Law, Establishing the European Food Safety Authority and Laying down Procedures in Matters of Food Safety. *Official Journal of the European Union.*

Regulation (EC) No 852/2004 of the European parliament and the council of 29 April 2004 on the hygiene of foodstuffs. *Official Journal of the European Union.*

Regulation (EC) No 853/2004 of the European Parliament and of the Council of 29 April 2004 laying down specific hygiene rules for food of animal origin. *Official Journal of the European Union.*

Regulation (EC) No 854/2004 of the European Parliament and of the Council of 29 April 2004 laying down specific rules for the organisation of official controls on products of animal origin intended for human consumption. *Official Journal of the European Union.*

Regulation (EC) No 882/2004 of the European Parliament and of the Council of 29 April 2004 on official controls performed to ensure the verification of compliance with feed and food law, animal health and animal welfare rules. *Official Journal of the European Union.*

Regulation (EC) No 2073/2005 of the European parliament and the council of 15 November 2005 on microbiological criteria for foodstuffs. *Official Journal of the European Union.*

Regulation (EC) No 1441/2007 of the European parliament and the council of 5 December 2007 amending Regulation (EC) No 2073/2005 on microbiological criteria for foodstuffs. *Official Journal of the European Union.*

Sofos, J. N., 2008. Challenges to meat safety in the 21st century. *Meat Sci.,* 78, 3–13.

WHO, 2011. *Campylobacter.* Fact Sheet, No. 255.

Whyte, R., Hudson, J. A., Graham, C., 2006. *Campylobacter* in chicken livers and their destruction by pan frying. *Lett. Appl. Microbiol.*, 43, 591–595.

In: Campylobacter Infections
Editor: Brittany A. Bertucci
ISBN: 978-1-63463-858-6

Chapter 4

Virulence and Adaptation Strategies of *Campylobacter* spp. and Its Relationship to Clinical Disease

Roberta Torres de Melo*[*], *Eliane Pereira Mendonça, Guilherme Paz Monteiro, Belchiolina Beatriz Fonseca, and Daise Aparecida Rossi
Laboratory of Applied Animal Biotechnology and
Laboratory of Molecular Epidemiology,
Faculty of Veterinary Medicine - Federal University of Uberlândia, Brazil

Abstract

The infection by *Campylobacter* spp. constitutes a worldwide distribution of zoonosis, with serious repercussions for public health and a significant socio-economic impact. Representatives of this genus are the most common etiologic agents of gastroenteritis caused by food. *C. jejuni* and *C. coli* are recognized as the most important species and with greater pathogenic potential from the food safety's point of view. The raw milk consumption, non-potable water, and other food of animal origin might be the source of human infection. However, poultry is an important

[*] Corresponding author: Email: roberta-melo@hotmail.com.

reservoir of *Campylobacter*, thus becomes the main target of control measures. Understanding the epidemiology of *Campylobacter* and the main challenges in its control, contributes to determine the risk posed to human health. The difficulty of isolating and cultivating *Campylobacter;* and the high cost, results in a lack of accurate data in the diseases' occurrence in the world. It is known that despite the apparent *Campylobacter*'s fragility to the environmental conditions, this agent is able to create mechanisms that allow their metabolic adaptation and growth change quickly in different environmental conditions in which they are submitted. This ability allows the detection of different behaviors that can explain their ability to survive and multiply in stressful conditions. These parameters directly affect the prevalence and persistence of *Campylobacter* in food destined for consumption. The epidemiology of infections caused by *Campylobacter* spp. are considered complex, presenting multiple determinants in this microorganism spread. Among these factors, are represented important virulence factors in the agent's pathogenesis, resulting in greater severity of clinical disease. The infection by *Campylobacter* causes gastroenteritis in humans and takes place orally through contact with infected animals as domestic or production animal, and food consumption, which is the most important pathway. The clinical manifestation of the disease can have from mild to severe symptoms, including watery diarrhea (sometimes with blood), abdominal pain, fever, headache, nausea and to progressive paralysis that can result in respiratory failure and severe neurological dysfunction and may even lead to death. The occurrence of campylobacteriosis outbreaks requires immediate notification to the surveillance authorities, in order to initiate the investigation of common sources and transmission control through preventive measures, thereby minimizing the potential risks to human health.

Introduction

The microbiological quality of the food produced in a country or imported, is one of the pillars for ensuring the public health. Outbreaks of foodborne diseases cause direct and indirect damages, endangering the health of consumers and have an impact on the economy. Among the microorganisms, most incriminated in food outbreaks, the genus *Campylobacter* (Scientific Status Summary, 2004; EFSA, 2009) stands out.

The reservoir of these microorganisms is the intestinal tract of domestic, wild or production animals; which are mainly chickens (Moore et al., 2005; Keller et al., 2007).

Campylobacter spp. is recognized worldwide as the principal bacteria that causes diarrhea in humans and is reported as the most common zoonotic infection (Moore et al., 2005; EFSA, 2009).

Between the species involved in gastroenteric diseases, C. jejuni is the most prevalent (Hirsh, 2003). Although it is self-limiting in healthy adults, children, elderly or immunocompromised individuals can become a severe disease requiring antibiotic therapy. However, in most cases occur individual sporadic infections (Cox, 2002). Humans become infected by direct contact with carrier animals; eating raw or undercooked meat of poultry, pork, and cattle; by ingestion of unpasteurized milk and water (FDA, 2008).

The gastroenteritis caused by Campylobacter spp. in humans is characterized by profuse diarrhea, acute abdominal pain and fever. In a small percentage of cases, this infection can lead to potentially serious complications (Lastovica, 2006), such as Guillain-Barré Syndrome (GBS), a disorder resulting in acute neuromuscular paralysis. It is estimated that approximately one in every 1,000 *Campylobacter* infections leads to GBS (Pope et al., 2007; Rabinstein, 2007).

Besides the agent's identification, it is also important to know the intrinsic characteristics of these microorganisms, since it's able to cause disease by strains of *Campylobacter* species; it is not homogeneous and it is related to virulence factors. Thus, the use of these markers associated with human diarrheal disease factors, the processes of cell invasion, the mechanisms of resistance to stressful conditions and neurological syndromes; have demonstrated the degree of virulence of strains present in food products and the hazards to the consumer (Habib et al., 2012).

Characterization of *Campylobacter* spp. Responsible for Gastroenteritis

Among the species and subspecies of *Campylobacter* that have already been identified, the most important are those which belong to the thermophilic group, particularly *Campylobacter jejuni*, *Campylobacter coli* and *Campylobacter lari*, where the first two are the species which are more frequently isolated in case of gastroenteritis in humans and animals (Center for Food Security & Public Health [CFSPH], 2005).

These bacteria are thermophilic with optimal growth between 37-42 °C and microaerophilic (Silva= et al., 2011). However, *C. jejuni* is able to survive in environments with temperatures of 27 °C with 60% to 62% relative humidity (Davis; Conner, 2007). The metabolic activity of these microorganisms does not cease at low temperatures, because they develop mechanisms of environmental adaptation, allowing their residence to process at 4 °C or under freezing foods (Ligowska et al., 2011; Melo, 2012).

It may also contribute to its permanence in the environment and the consequent high number of infections. The fact that when they are in unfavorable conditions of development a cytoplasmic retraction can occur, in which cells pass into a coccoid form. This condition can occur by aging the cultures (more than 48 hours), oxidative or thermal stress. This gives the bacteria the ability to enter a state that can be described as "viable non culturable" (VNC), which allows you to survive the changes of environmental stress and even uncultivable in culture media, remaining infective in order to maintain its virulence. When environmental conditions become favorable again, it is possible to reverse to the spiral shape and the multiplication (Il-Keum et al., 2007).

These agents are classified as fastidious and that is why *Campylobacter* is difficult to isolate, identify and cultivate (WHO, 2013). The detection in food must be taken into account the fact that the population in the products is usually low due to no growth at temperatures below 30 °C and extreme sensitivity to the oxygen concentration of air (21%). Success usually depends on the detection analysis of a large number of samples, concentration of present cells and enrichment under microaerophilic conditions at a temperature of 42 °C (Silva et al., 1997).

Epidemiological Aspects

According to CDC (2012), in the United States of America, *Campylobacter* is the leading cause of bacterial diarrhea, with one million documented cases occurring annually as mostly isolated and sporadic events. 90% of these cases are associated to the *Campylobacter jejuni* species and the remaining is assigned to *Campylobacter coli*.

The seasonality can affect the incidence and/or prevalence of human campylobacteriosis, and sporadic cases, which constitute the majority of the most common infections in the summer, are often underappreciated. These sporadic cases are assigned to the handling and consumption of raw or poorly processed poultry, as well as cross-contamination that may occur during the simultaneous handling of poultry meat and raw foods (Jore et al., 2010).

According to the Report of the EFSA (2009), the highest number of campylobacteriosis cases in humans is reported during the summer months. However, some studies show the presence of the monthly peaks because of the seasonal trends (Habib et al., 2012; Melo, 2012).

The main risk factor for human of acquiring campylobacteriosis is related to alimentation and the handling of poultry; mainly raw or poorly processed chicken, accounting for 50% to 70% of the cases (Sermiene; Malakauskas, 2008). This contamination can occur throughout the production chain, either directly or indirectly by cross-contamination, that poses a major risk to human health (Ellis-Iversen et al., 2009).

Campylobacter has high survivability in extreme conditions during the production process of chickens due to the ability of fixation in feather follicles and deep cracks in the bird's skin. These recesses provide ideal conditions for the bacteria to adhere and support the variations in processing conditions (Jang et al., 2007).

These data corroborate a study conducted in Belgium, which revealed that the prevalence of *Campylobacter* in broiler flocks and on their carcasses is quite high and equivalent to 41.1% and 45.9% (Botteldoorn et al., 2008). The same was observed in a study conducted in Ireland in 2008, in which 394 of broiler chilled carcasses studied, 98% were contaminated with *C. jejuni* (EFSA, 2010). In some member countries of the European Union (EU) in 2007, the prevalence of fresh chicken meat was equivalent to 83%. In Iran, the prevalence was 63% and in Japan was 45.8% (FAO, 2009).

In Brazil, Melo (2012) isolated *Campylobacter* spp. in 22.38% of 420 chilled and frozen chicken carcasses produced in slaughterhouses of three different Brazilian southeastern and central-western states. A lower rate of contamination than obtained by Kuana et al. (2008), who obtained results equivalent to 99% of the chilled carcasses contaminated with *Campylobacter* spp. in the state of Rio Grande do Sul. Franchin et al. (2007) studied 335 samples of chilled carcasses, water and equipment collected at different points inside the broiler slaughter line in the state of Santa Catarina and they found positivity for *Campylobacter* in 71.3% of the samples.

In addition to chickens, *Campylobacter* can be found in cattle, pigs, turkeys, ducks, or lamb (Humphrey et al., 2007). In fact, the digestive tract of healthy cattle is an important reservoir for some species of *Campylobacter* (Atabay & Corry, 1998), the prevalence of which varies from 0 to 80%. In sheep, the prevalence is about 20% (Zwueifel & Stephan, 2004). In pork the prevalence of the agent is more often compared to beef or lamb (Nesbakken et al., 2003), which is because the swine carcasses are subjected to a common phase of scalding at the beginning of the slaughter process combined with the fact that the skin remains on the substrate throughout all the processing (Moore et al., 2005).

Contaminated shellfish have also been implicated as a vehicle for the transmission of campylobacteriosis. The existence of contaminated water with *Campylobacter* appears to be the most likely cause of infection (Moore & Wilson, 1996).

The consumption of untreated water (Schorr et al., 1994) has also been considered as a risk factor for infection. In a study conducted in Sweden, positive associations were found between the incidence of *Campylobacter* spp. and water consumption, which can be directly related to the proportion of sporadic cases of human campylobacteriosis (Nygard et al., 2004).

Milk was also identified as a vehicle for human gastroenteritis caused by *Campylobacter* spp. (Potter et al., 1983). The agent's survival in this food matrix has been characterized as an important risk factor in the transmission of microorganism (Monteiro, 2013). *C. jejuni* can be present in the milk, due to cross-contamination with feces during milking, or as a result of udder infection, besides handling it in places where there is presence of animal products origin (Orr et al., 1995; EFSA, 2013).

Besides the risk of acquiring campylobacteriosis via food and water consumption, contact with the animals, both, domestic and livestock represents another route of exposure to human infection (Andersson, 2000; Roberts, 2011). The environmental contamination by feces of domestic and wild animals is an additional risk for infection (Said et al., 2003).

Humans may also contributes to the spread of the agent primarily by the fecal-oral route, since infected may continue to excrete the microorganism on average of two to three weeks after clinical recovery, when there is no treatment with antimicrobials (Sallam, 2007).

Among the determinants factors of high prevalence of campylobacteriosis in humans, probably the low infective dose of the agent is an aggravating factor. The infective *Campylobacter*'s dose is only about 400 to 500 cells (Amri et al., 2007).

Despite all the available studies on *Campylobacter* spp., the epidemiology of this agent is complex and still not fully understood. Many countries, especially developing ones, still do not know the real incidence of infections by this agent, further studies on the importance of different sources of infection and the role of the host is required (Ridley et al., 2008).

Clinical Manifestations of the Disease

According to World Health Organization (WHO, 2011), *Campylobacter* is the main cause of severe cases of diarrhea, however, people mostly present recovery in a period from two to five days, although it can last up to 10 days. Rarely the infection results in consequences that remain for a long period, resulting in more complicated diseases such as, sepsis, abortion, meningitis, abscesses and complications like Guillain-Barré Syndrome.

The Guillain-Barré Syndrome (SGB) is an autoimmune disease that causes generalized facial paralysis and annually may affect up to four people for every 100,000 inhabitants. Approximately 60% to 70% of patients with GBS have any acute illness of one to three weeks before symptoms appear, being most frequently infected by *Campylobacter jejuni*. This syndrome has a variant known as the Miller-Fisher Syndrome, which is characterized by ataxia, areflexia the ophthalmoplegia (BRAZIL, 2009).

SGB stands out as the most common cause of acute neuromuscular paralysis in the world. This syndrome is characterized as an autoimmune disease and a post-infectious with destruction of the myelin sheath of peripheral nerves, causing acute neuromuscular paralysis, which may compromise the breathing muscles and lead the patient to death (Kiernan, 2009).

When *C. jejuni* invades the human body, the immune response is the production of specific antibodies to the structure of its lipo-oligosaccharides. However, the human body contains compounds with exactly the same molecular structure and is found in the cell membrane of human nerve cells. Thus, the structure of the lipo-oligosaccharide of *C. jejuni* molecular structure mimics ganglioside and produced antibodies in response to the C. jejuni cell membrane also react against the nerve cell membrane. The result is damage, which occurs in nerve paralysis characteristic of Guillain-Barré Syndrome (Murray, 2007).

Another Syndrome resulting from infection by *Campylobacter jejuni* is Reiter's Syndrome and reactive arthritis. This syndrome is an autoimmune response that causes inflammation in different joints (arthritis) in response to infection by *C. jejuni*. It is more frequent in large weight-bearing joints such as the knees and lower back, but also other joints may be affected (Murray, 2007).

Among the common signs and symptoms in campylobacteriosis can be cited from aqueous, moderate and self-limiting diarrhea to a bloody dysentery; mucus with white blood cells, which may be accompanied by headaches, abdominal pain, fever, malaise, nausea, and vomiting. This condition is similar to those caused by many other enteric pathogenic microorganisms.

The phases of acute diarrhea lasts up to three days, but abdominal pain may persist for up to three weeks. The recovery is rapid and it takes generally a week. Antibiotic treatment is recommended only in severe cases. Repose and fluid therapy are indicated to reverse most of the symptoms, which in most cases are self-limiting (Sallam, 2007).

However, in some cases, *Campylobacter* species may cause some complications and long-term sequelae observed after classical manifestation of campylobacteriosis. These sequelae includes gastrointestinal, rheumatologic (Reiter's Syndrome), pulmonary, dermatological, intravascular, renal, neurological and abortive problems (Crushell et al., 2004).

Determinants of Pathogenicity

To establish a sufficient condition to cause infection, the microorganism must survive the physiological stress associated with internal and external environments such as temperature fluctuations, pH variations, and different types of hosts, host immunity, oxidative stress and limited supply of nutrients. Like all enteropathogenic bacteria, the genus *Campylobacter* evolved its attributes, many of which are virulence determinants that have helped circumvent the defenses of the human host, besides other hosts such as mammals and birds (Guerry, 2007).

Since the completion of the first genome project of *C. jejuni* (Parkhill et al., 2000), the mechanisms involved in the pathogenesis of this agent are still being unraveled. Molecular investigations of these mechanisms gained momentum and the knowledge of virulence determinants used by this microorganism persisting in the environment, surviving the acidity of the stomach and colonizing the intestinal epithelium is becoming clearer (Snelling et al., 2005).

For *C. jejuni* to develop in a sufficient level to cause disease infections is required to survive the physiological stresses associated with the external and internal environments, such as changes of temperature and pH in different hosts, in addition to oxidative stress and nutrient limitation (Snelling et al., 2005).

The most important virulence factors that designates this as a human pathogen agent includes: motility, chemotaxis, iron acquisition, adhesion, invasion, quorum sensing, defense to heat stress, response to heat stress, ability to form and avoid biofilms in the host's immune system. Other possible virulence factors include the production of toxin CDT and virulence plasmid, associated with the expression of *pVir* found in some strains of *C. jejuni* (Schmidt-Ott et al., 2005)

Motility

The polar flagellum was the first well-characterized outer structure of *C. jejuni* and represents one of the most important virulence factors involved in its pathogenesis. Besides allowing rapid mobility it acts as an adhesin, which helps in adhesion and invasion. Being intact and functional is essential to achieve optimal motility and allows colonization, which is critical to the development of the disease (Guerry et al., 2000a).

It is believed that both, the presence of flagella and the shape of corkscrews of *Campylobacters* contribute to its ability to remain in viscous environments such as the intestinal mucus. This ability is not found in other flagellated bacteria (Zilbauer et al., 2008).

The flagella of *C. jejuni* consist of three main components: the basal body, hook and filament. The filament consists of two flagellin proteins: the increased gene is encoded with *flaA* and *flaB* a lower encoding of the gene (Konkel et al., 2004). The expression of both genes ensures maximum potential virulence. The *flaA* gene indicates the absence of low mobility and reduction in flagellum's size, since the mutation in *flaB* is related to the presence of flagella in almost normal length and slightly lower motility, but it indicates a reduction in pathogenic potential (Wassenaar et al., 1993).

C. jejuni also demonstrates the ability to move in a reversible way and apparently spontaneously, between flagellates and non-flagellated phenotypes. This ability to modulate the flagellar expression is understandable with regard to energy cost for the expression and the need to adapt to environmental changes encountered during infection of a host and exposure to the external environment (Blackwell, 2010).

Besides motility, the flagellum also plays important roles in chemotaxis, colonization, biofilm formation and in the evasion of the innate immune response (Malik-Kale, 2008).

Chemotaxis

The chemotaxis' mechanisms make the microorganism moves toward opposite direction of the chemical stimulus. Thus, the chemotactic response of *C. jejuni* is important for the pathogen to target specific sites in which are favorable for the development and multiplication in the intestinal tract as well as away from adverse environments (Konkel, 2001).

The bacterial chemotaxis is a complex signal transduction system by which bacteria are able to recognize and respond to environmental stimuli with flagellar rotation (Marchant et al., 2002). Thus, when the receiver detects an increase in the concentration of attractive stimuli in the environment; bacteria remain moving freely, or when detecting a reduction in the concentration of the stimulus, the bacteria change direction to get to a favorable environment (Bhavsar & Kapadnis, 2007).

The pathogenic mechanism of this expression is made potential at 37 °C, which is the physiological temperature of humans (Khanna et.al, 2006).

In addition to the optimum temperature found in the human host, *Campylobacter* jejuni uses a component of the mucin present in the intestinal mucus, L-fucose, as a source of energy and multiplication. This metabolic substrate facilitates adaptation in environments with low nutrient levels, which provides a competitive advantage to that organism (Muraoka & Zhang, 2011).

Both motility and chemotaxis have an important role in virulence and host colonization. Chemotaxis is required for optimal recognition sites for invasion of host tissues and through the motility; the agent is able to move in favor of chemical gradient, which presents optimal conditions for colonization (Snelling et al., 2005). The sequence of the *C. jejuni* genome revealed the presence of several genes involved in chemotaxis, as *che* and *aer* (Korolik & Ketley, 2005).

Still much has to be understood in terms of how all the elements combine to chemotactic control of motility and behavior of *C. jejuni*. However, it is known that the chemotactic motility is essential for the survival of the host microorganism and it is a prerequisite to cause disease in humans (Dasti, 2010).

Adhesion

Adherence to epithelial cells of the gastrointestinal tract of the host is an important colonization factor for *Campylobacter jejuni*. The act of adhesion between micro-organisms and host cells is an essential first step in how this pathogen initiates infection (Feistel, 2011).

The contact of *C. jejuni* with the host epithelium causes damage to the intestinal epithelial cells, but does not deregulates the absorption function, as it happens with enteropathogens (Kopecko & Hu, 2000). This step is ensured by the presence of adhesins that are located in the flagella and other cell surface components such as, for example, the lipopolysaccharide (LPS) (Feistel, 2011).

Adhesins are macromolecules exposed on the cell's surface that facilitates the microorganism to bind to the host cell receptors (Chiapparrone et al., 2011). Some adhesins found in strains of *Campylobacter jejuni* include *CadF* (*Campylobacter* adhesion to fibronectin), capA (*Campylobacter* adhesion protein), *JlpA* (jejuni lipoprotein and PEB1 (Protein Pei) (Flanagan et al., 2009; Konkel et al., 2010). Other molecules also act as adhesins including flagella, the lipopolysaccharide (LPS) and the cap (CPS) (Konkel, 2001).

The *CadF* adhesin is one of the most important and this mechanism is required by *C. jejuni* for maximum adherence and invasion into intestinal epithelial cells of the host, being the adhesion of *CadF*, the first step to bacterial internalization (Monteville & Konkel 2002). This adhesin protein is a 37kDa outer membrane mainly found in *C. jejuni,* which binds specific receptors on the basolateral surface and maximizes the host cell invasion (Monteville et al., 2003). It binds fibronectin (Fn), which is a glycoprotein present in the junction regions of the gastrointestinal epithelial cells and provides a binding site with potential pathogens. The *CadF* connection promotes interaction between the pathogen and the host cell; permits translocation of bacteria retaining the intact epithelial barrier; and facilitating colonization by microorganism (Krause-Gruszczynska et al., 2007).

Invasion

After the colonization of the host cell, *Campylobacter jejuni* invades the intestinal cells. There is the participation of a CiaB protein (*Campylobacter* invasion antigens B) (Konkel, 2003) to get this result. The secretion of this protein requires an environmental stimulus such as the presence of bile salts on the environment of the host cell components and pathogen, such as flagella (Guerry, 2007).

The *ciaB* gene encodes the CiaB 73-kD protein, which is associated with the export mechanism of flagellin. This protein is linked to the destruction of the microtubule promoting mobility and allowing the entry of bacteria inside the host cell. The mechanism of invasion produced by CiaB induces disruption of microtubule motors and cellular microfilaments, besides tyrosine phosphorylation of cytoplasmic proteins, which are a signaling cascade of reactions, promoting cell disorders in order to enhance intracytoplasmic motility without restrictions (Ribera-Amill et al., 2001).

Another gene of great importance in the invasive process of *Campylobacter* is *pldA*. This gene encodes a protein involved in the synthesis of outer membrane phospholipase (Ziprin et al., 2001). Phospholipases are a subgroup of lipolytic enzymes which are capable of hydrolyzing one or more ester bonds in phospholipids promoting disruption of cell membrane in eukaryotes. The protein derived from *pldA* gene is located in the outer membrane of the bacteria and has hemolytic property and it can be responsible for tissue damage during infection by *C. jejuni* or *C. coli*. The absence of this gene in the expression promotes a significant reduction in haemolytic activity and ability to cecal colonization in chickens (Matoba et al., 2002).

The invasion occurs by endocytosis and starts with signaling in the host cell surface. This signal, which is associated with cytoplasmic proteins, is recognized by receptors present on the cell membrane. These proteins form depression in the outer membrane when the receivers are connected to microorganisms. This depression increases and becomes cytoplasmic vacuoles (Levin, 2007).

The infected epithelial cells exhibit swelling, loss of microvilli and premature apoptosis due to the cytotoxic effect of *C. jejuni* (Melo et al., 2013). Subsequently, the formed vacuole migrates to the own lamina and then *C. jejuni* is released along with the contents of the epithelial cell, triggering an inflammatory process (Levin, 2007).

The efficiency of *C. jejuni's* invasion is strain-dependent. Bacterial factors are known to play an important role in a cellular invasion including motility (flagellar apparatus) and adhesion (Malik-Kale, 2008). Moreover, it is associated with the cell type, as it seems to be more efficiently internalized in strains of human origin (Hu; Kopecko, 1999).

Thus, host factors are also involved in the invasion process. Among them, we highlight the cytoskeleton comprising microtubules (MT) and microfilaments (MF) that are directly involved in the absorption of *Campylobacter* (Fonseca, 2011). The alteration of this structure by *C. jejuni* is mediated by proteins Cdc42 and Rac1, which act as molecular switches and alter the signal transduction of the host, causing polymerization and rearrangement of microfilaments and microtubules; and facilitating internalization (Gruszczynska-Krause et al., 2007).

Despite the various studies related to the invasion process, the exact molecular mechanisms involved in this step of *C. jejuni* infection are not yet completely understood (Lodge, 2007).

Toxins

Although the invasion of *Campylobacter spp.* is sufficient to cause disease, the production of toxins also contributes to the development of campylobacteriosis (Ge et al., 2008). The cytopathic effects that are observed in enteritis are caused not only by the invasion process, but also because of the action of enterotoxins and/or cytotoxins (Zilbauer et al., 2008).

Cytotoxins are defined as proteins which cause the death of the target cells. They act by inhibiting essential cellular processes, for example, protein synthesis, formation of actin filaments and the formation of pores in the membrane of target cells, resulting in cell death by lysis (Abuoun et al., 2005).

The extensional cytolethal toxin (CDT) is the most important one and it is encoded by three genes, *cdtA*, *cdtB* and *cdtC*. All three must be expressed to a fully cytotoxic action. The proteins of the *cdtA* and *cdtC* genes function in the transport of CdtB protein that is internalized by the host cell. Within the cell, the CdtB protein enhances the obstruction of the cell cycle, by exhibiting a similar activity to DNase, resulting in cuts in double-stranded DNA. Host cells respond to DNA cuts, blocking the G2 phase of mitotic division, inducing a cytoplasmic strain that leads to cell death by apoptosis in about three to four days after infection (Asakura et al., 2007; Melo et al., 2013).

The CDT activity may differ slightly depending on the affected cell lineage. The pathogenic mechanism of CDT is related to the inhibition of humoral and cellular immunity via apoptosis of immune cells; it can cause necrosis of the epithelial and fibroblast cells involved in repair of lesions produced by the pathogen, resulting in a slow healing and induction of the disease's symptoms. Therefore, it interferes in the division and differentiation of cells of the intestinal crypts, contributing to the development of diarrhea (Smith; Bayles, 2006).

Probably there is a relationship between the toxin in watery diarrhea symptoms and a reduction in the function of normal absorption. However, the role of CDT in the pathogenesis of *C. jejuni* is not yet well understood (AbuOun et al., 2005).

Adaption Strategies

Campylobacter jejuni is able to colonize many different hosts and compete against the intestinal microbiota. To do this, the agent must be able to efficiently acquire a sufficient amount of nutrients and have adaptive strategies to assist in their survival and growth (Stahl et al., 2012).

To be successful, *C. jejuni* must have the ability to survive in a wide variety of hosts, such as humans and animals; different environments, in addition to water and food. This requires some degrees of adaptive flexibility, which is indicated as impressive for this specie considering the relatively small number of different metabolic pathways identified in their genome (Stahl et al., 2012).

Endosymbiosis with Amoebae

It is important to highlight that some bacterial species require special growing conditions, such as *C. jejuni* that can survive and even multiply within free-living amoebae, establishing endosymbiotic relationships (Axelsson-Olsson et al., 2005; Olofsson et al., 2013). This kind of symbiosis between bacteria and protozoa, especially with *Acanthamoeba castellanii*, has also been described by Arcobacter butzleri, specie of the family Campylobacteraceae (Fernandez et al., 2012; Medina et al., 2014).

The fact that *C. jejuni* survives within free-living amoebae, can have serious repercussions epidemiologically because these protozoa may act as reservoirs and/or vectors of bacteria that have the ability to survive as endosymbionts (Greub and Raoult, 2004; Khan, 2006). Furthermore, amoebas protect any microorganism that is inside due to resisting the action of disinfectants and adverse environmental conditions (King et al., 1988; Price Kilvington, 1990; Barker et al., 1992).

Regarding this fact, it has been shown that free-living amoebae can inhabit water systems and even those that used treatments in water; drastically reduce the number of amoeba. This protozoa can propagate to these distribution networks despite the existence of processes of disinfection using ozone and chlorine (Hoffmann and Michel, 2001; Corsaro et al., 2008; Thomas et al., 2008), which could be considered as an important mechanism for the dissemination of endosymbiotic bacterias with free-living amoebae, as *Campylobacter spp.*

Endosymbiosis of *Campylobacter spp.* within free-living amoebae does not only have epidemiological consequences that directly affect humans. In 2005, it was established that the failure to reduce contamination of poultry may be due to the part of the ability of *C. jejuni* to resist the disinfection of potable water intended for birds, due to their ability to internalize in waterborne protozoa. The results of this research means that those protozoas in potable water of chickens destined for human consumption may delay the decrease of viability of *Campylobacter spp.* and increase the disinfection resistance of these bacteria, thereby increasing the possibility that the chickens are colonized by them (Snelling et al., 2005)

Antimicrobial Resistance

The introduction of antimicrobial agents in clinical practice of human and animal medicine is one of the greatest achievements of the health sector. However, the indiscriminate or inappropriate use can contribute to the emergence of antimicrobial resistance. Antimicrobial resistance is recognized by the World Health Organization (WHO) as one of the major public health concern, since it is a problem of global dimensions (Moore et al., 2006).

According Aarestrup (2005), a wide variety of antimicrobials is used in animal production. They can be administered both in treatment and in prevention of disease; and as growth promoters, resulting in increased feed efficiency and actual weight gain. However, most of these drugs are used in subtherapeutic doses, which favor the selection, multiplication and persistence of resistant bacterial strains.

Campylobacter spp. and other bacteria can become a potential reservoir of resistance genes that can be transmitted horizontally to other pathogenic bacteria. For this reason, the antimicrobial resistance of commensal bacteria of the gastrointestinal tract is an indication of selective pressure by use of these drugs. In addition, antimicrobial agents may remain as waste products of animal origin, which allows a selection of resistant bacteria after the consumption of such food, or may be discharged to the environment in the form of human or animal effluents (Fabrega et al., 2008).

Infections caused by *Campylobacter spp.* are usually self-limiting and treated primarily with fluid therapy; in some cases the use of antimicrobial agents is required. According to Han et al. (2007), macrolides and fluoroquinolones are the drugs of choice in the treatment of campylobacteriosis. Tetracycline is cited as an alternative treatment and in the case of more serious infections, such as bacteremia and sepsis, intravenous aminoglycosides are administered.

However, it has been reported that the rates of antibiotic resistance in bacteria isolated from humans, especially to fluoroquinolones, have risen sharply in the last 20 years and these high rates of resistance are seen today in many regions of the world (CDC, 2013b).

Knowing that campylobacteriosis is transmitted by the consumption of food, the use of antibiotics in the different stages of the poultry production chain can promote or assist the spread of resistant strains. Various reports around the world associated infections with *Campylobacter spp.* resistant to fluoroquinolones with the approval of the use of antimicrobials in poultry production (Engberg et al., 2001; Ge et al. 2003; Gupta et al., 2004; Kinana et al. 2006; Serichantalergs et al., 2007). To tackle the emergence of fluoroquinolone-resistant strains in the United States, the Food and Drug Administration (FDA) withdrew its approval for the use of fluoroquinolones in poultry since 2005 (Zhao et al., 2010).

Patterns of antimicrobial use and resistance selection in one part of the world also affects other regions, since there is entrainment of agents in international travel and the food trade, constituting another aggravating factor for the spread of resistance to these drugs profiles. It has been noted that the fluoroquinolone-resistant infections are often associated with travel to developed or developing countries (Hakanen et al., 2003; Kassenborg et al., 2004). The most comprehensive collection of such information may provide a way to monitor resistance patterns in parts of the world where local surveillance is limited or nonexistent. It is difficult to perform systematic studies of control cases among travelers, but comparison of these strains isolated from persons with meat, poultry or other food products imported from these countries can be useful. This information is of particular value when combined with detailed reports about the use of antimicrobials in animal and human data. Data on the prevalence of resistance should be the starting point in assessing the risk associated with antimicrobial resistance (WHO, 2011).

In the US, in 2010, 1% of *C. jejuni* isolates from humans were resistant to erythromycin (macrolide), 43% to tetracycline (tetracycline) and 22% to ciprofloxacin (fluoroquinolone) (CDC, 2012). The comparable values were 1% to erythromycin, 36% to tetracycline and 22% to ciprofloxacin (FDA, 2011) of *C. jejuni* isolates from broiler meat. In the European Union, also in 2010, 2% of *C. jejuni* isolates from humans were resistant to erythromycin, 21% to tetracycline and 52% to fluoroquinolones. The numbers were respectively 2%, 22% and 50% (EFSA, 2012) found in chicken meat.

Considering the data of the US and EU resistance, the resistance was generally greater in *C. coli* than *C. jejuni* (CDC, 2012; EFSA, 2012). A study conducted in the EU in 2011, showed slightly higher rates to those found in 2010. In *Campylobacter* isolated from humans, resistance levels were higher for nalidixic acid (47.8%) and ciprofloxacin (44.4 %), followed by ampicillin (35.3%) and tetracycline (30.5%). Low levels of resistance were observed for clinically importance in the treatment of campylobacteriosis with erythromycin (average of 3.5%). Multidrug resistance in human isolates was high or very high in some European countries (EFSA, 2013b).

Also in Europe, resistance was extremely high to ciprofloxacin (fluoroquinolone) commonly observed in *C. coli* isolates from broiler and chicken meat (76.6% and 77.7%, respectively), with slightly lower levels in *C. jejuni* (57.2% and 59.2%, respectively). High values were also reported in isolates from pigs and cattle (35.5% and 38.8%). Important differences between animal species and sites of isolation were observed. Resistance to erythromycin was detected in low percentages in *Campylobacter spp.* isolates from broiler and chicken meat (1.6% and 9.8%), with the exception of *C. coli*, in which was a moderate resistance (15.5 %) detected. The highest level of erythromycin resistance was observed in *C. coli* isolates from pigs (24.5%), while in cattle *C. jejuni* isolates were very low (0.8%). Resistance to nalidixic acid was common among *Campylobacter spp.* isolates from meat and animals (32.4% and 74.6%). The multidrug resistance (resistance to at least three classes of antibiotics according to epidemiological cutoff values) was generally low in *C. jejuni* isolates from chicken and chicken meat, and the co-resistance to clinically important antibiotics, ciprofloxacin and erythromycin was in the same isolates, nor recorded or detected at low levels. Levels of multidrug resistance and co-resistance were generally higher in *C. coli* isolates from broiler chickens (EFSA, 2013b).

Melo (2012), when analyzing *Campylobacter spp.* isolates from frozen and refrigerated broiler carcasses from the states of Minas Gerais, Distrito Federal and Goiás in Brazil, found 43.6% of resistance to norfloxacin (fluoroquinolone), 36.2% to erythromycin (macrolides), and 34.0 % to tetracycline. It also determined that the joint resistance to macrolide and fluoroquinolone was a characteristic shared by 19.1% (18/94) of the strains, being six *C. jejuni*, six *C. coli* and six *Campylobacter spp.*

Iron Acquisition

Iron is an essential nutrient for bacterial growth and survival, as it plays an important role in many biochemical reactions catalysis that are required for almost all living organisms. It is an important co-factor in DNA synthesis and reactions requiring transfer of electrons, however, their purchase from the environment presents a problem, since the free iron is almost nonexistent (Miller et al., 2009).

As a result, bacteria have had to develop ways to acquire iron from their environment, although too much iron can be harmful. In the presence of oxygen, iron can cause the generation of oxygen's free radicals, which can damage the DNA, proteins and membranes. For this reason, the iron storage systems and strategies to combat the effects of oxidative stress are also important for bacterial survival *in vivo*. After the process of intestinal colonization, it is essential that *C. jejuni* is able to effectively compete with the intestinal microbiota by the acquisition of iron to maintain sufficient amounts of this element from the host to its growth and avoid accumulating because of the toxic potential (Lodge, 2007).

Several iron uptake systems have been described for *C. jejuni*: siderophore (enterochelin, ferrichrome and rodotorulic acid) absorption from sources of iron (heme group and transferrin protein), transduction systems and absorption of ferrous iron (Miller et al., 2009).

The *p19* gene encodes a periplasmic protein (permease) with a size of 19kDa iron-dependent, whose function is to transport iron (Miller et al., 2009). The regulation of this protein indicates a way to control the level of intracellular element during stress and its absence is associated with the inability to use iron as rodotoluric acid blocking the growth (Birk, 2012).

The requirement of iron uptake systems, as conferred by the P19 protein for successful host colonization emphasizes the need for detailed studies of molecular characterization on different isolates of *C. jejuni* (Miller et al., 2009).

Tolerance to Low Temperatures

The freezing process of the bacterial cells induces stress due to intracellular dehydration. It is proven that some of the damage caused by cooling results in the release of superoxide radicals. Therefore, the expression of SOD proteins (superoxide dismutase) present in situations of stress, aids in the survival of *C. jejuni* under freezing conditions (Stead and Park, 2000).

The production of enzymes such as superoxide dismutase (SODs) was shown to be important virulence factors for *Campylobacter spp*. Three types of SODs enzymes have been described: cofactors that contain iron (sodB or FeSOD), manganese (sodA or MnSOD), copper and zinc (sodC CuZnSOD). These enzymes catalyze the breakdown of superoxide molecules into hydrogen peroxide and dioxygen. Thus, constitute a major mechanism of cell defense against oxidative stress (Hassan, 1988). The increased expression of SOD by stress caused by low temperatures is related to the protection of cellular components, including various cytoplasmic enzymes, DNA, and membrane factors (Stintzi & Whitworth, 2003).

Tolerance to low temperatures in *Campylobacter* species is strain-dependent. Furthermore, the maintenance of micro-organisms under these extreme conditions does not favor the formation of viable culturable cells (VNC), which reduces the transcription process of virulence characteristics (Moura, 2013). However, the return to cultivable state can be reestablished by a passage through a host (Sampers et al., 2009).

Dimitraki & Velonakis (2007) point out that freezing inhibits growth of *Campylobacter*, reduce their numbers but did not eliminate them completely in frozen foods, such as chicken meat (Humphrey et al., 2007). The survivability of *Campylobacter spp.* in extreme condition during the cycle of broiler production can be associated with the ability of fixing the deep crevices of the chicken's skin. These recesses provide ideal conditions for bacteria to adhere and to support the changes in conditions during processing (Lee et al., 1998). Jang et al. (2007) demonstrated that cells of *Campylobacter* could not only persists in the feathers follicles, but also be able to penetrate the skin and be protected by keeping the spiral shape.

The constitution of the surface of chicken also assists in survival of *C. jejuni* at 5 °C, compared with culture media in the laboratory. This is probably explained by the present compounds in chicken influencing in any way, the adaptation of the microorganism at low temperatures as well as the transcription of genes associated with prolonged survival of *C. jejuni* (Ligowska et al., 2011).

In addition, *Campylobacter* presents mechanisms of tolerance and adaptation to low temperatures including the acquisition or biosynthesis of cryoprotectant molecules, leading to changes in the lipid composition of the membrane in order to keep it viable under these conditions (Stintzi & Whitworth, 2003).

Tolerance to High Temperatures

C. jejui is exposed to multiple stresses during production of animal origin food and it is still able to survive in the final product. This adaptation allows the potential for pathogens withstand different stress conditions, including tolerance to high temperatures. These are phenomena known as specific adaptive response or multiple adaptive response or cross-protection (Isohanni et al., 2013;. Xu et al., 2008).

Despite the high temperatures encountered during slaughter of poultry, *C. jejuni* provides support mechanisms to heat stress. And these are expressed more efficiently when the strain is subjected to nutrient scarcity and stress caused by reduced pH (Klančnik et al., 2009; Reid et al., 2008).

The thermoregulation plays an important role in the expression of virulence genes in pathogenic bacteria, including *C. jejuni*. The microorganisms respond to heat stress by inducing the synthesis of a highly conserved group of proteins, whose synthesis rate varies with temperature, but rapidly increases after a sudden rise in temperature or in response to other environmental stresses (Reid et al. 2008). Already during the stress by cold shock, the genes of protein translation of heat shock repress their expression (Beales, 2004). Besides playing important roles in thermotolerance and dealing with other physiological stresses, gene transcription, such as *dnaJ*, is essential for normal functioning of cells.

The *dnaJ* gene expression indicates that the strain encodes a heat shock protein which allows the bacteria to grow in the upper temperature at 40 °C and is thermotolerant (Konkel et al., 1998). Proteins derived from the *dnaJ* gene have an important role in overcoming rapid changes in temperature, so the microorganism becomes able to survive and adapt to the new temperature (Stintzi, 2003). The heat shock response is also associated with the development of intestinal tract's colonization and bacteria survival in high temperatures (Konkel et al., 1998).

Furthermore, the adaptive processes involving the thermal shock tolerance also help in protecting periplasmic proteins that act in the transport of nutrients, in the glycosylation of proteins and the respiration process (Miller et al., 2009). These proteins are constantly exposed to thermal variations and thus can suffer deformations which prevent the execution of vital processes to *C. jejuni*. Thus, the expression of genes such as *dnaJ*, *dnaK* and *htrA* is important to degrade deformed or damaged proteins, promoting proper conformation of the protein and protect it from changes that lead to denaturation (Bæk et al., 2011).

Quorum-Sensing Mechanism

Several bacterial mechanisms of intercellular communication have been identified in a wide range of species. These systems are collectively called *quorum-sensing* (QS) and play important roles in a variety of physiological processes including motility, biofilm formation, the expression of virulence genes and animal colonization (Plummer, 2012).

Quorum-sensing (QS) refers to the phenomenon of cell-cell communication between bacteria. This mechanism is dependent on the release of signaling molecules called autoinducers (AIs). When the concentration of AIs reaches a certain threshold, the microorganisms are able to coordinate their behavior by regulating gene expression, and thus control the bacterial phenotype and initiate a response to the population level (Bandara et al., 2012).

This system is associated with a variety of interactive social responses by bacteria, including virulence, antimicrobial resistance, maintenance and maturation of the biofilm, motility, symbiosis, aggregation, conjugal plasmid transfer, production of toxins, bioluminescence and establish an infection (Bandara et al., 2012). The latter is associated with the locking activation of the mechanisms in the presence of the pathogen until they have a sufficient number of bacteria to establish infection (Jayaraman & Wood, 2008).

Varieties of QS systems have been detected both in Gram-negative as Gram-positive bacteria. The first evidence came from the study of bacterial communication dependent bioluminescence in *Vibrio fischeri* density. The induction of bioluminescence is mediated by dependent action of small concentrations of signaling compounds produced by bacteria called autoinducers. This work has provided the basis for the model quorum-sensing in Gram-negative bacteria (Engebrecht & Silverman, 1984).

In *Campylobacter spp.*, there is production of AI-1 (acyl-homoserine autoinducer) which accumulates in extracellular medium and diffuses freely in the bacterial cytoplasm. When intracellular levels of AI reach a critical concentration limit, it binds to a cellular transcription activator (*luxS*) encoding luciferase (Bassler, 1999), featuring a key enzyme in the metabolic pathway for recycling SAM (S adenosylmethionine). This metabolite is essential in the performance of major biosynthetic reactions such as methylation of bacterial DNA synthesis and bacterial polyamine vitamins (Parveen and Cornell, 2011).

The most important role of *luxS* gene is associated with the synthesis of a new AI called autoinducer-2 (AI-2) (Rajan et al., 2005). The increased growth of the bacterial population also promotes high concentrations of AI-2 in the environment. The *luxS* gene acts in the formation of various molecular compounds variants that are termed together AI-2. These molecules have potential for recognition and inclusion of mixed populations of the same species (Xavier & Bassler, 2005a). However, there are also variations in cell recognition mechanism. Evidence shows that AI-2 may also send the signal from specie to make the response of other species (Holmes et al., 2009).

In addition to the dual function of LuxS both as a metabolic enzyme as one synthase precursor protein for IA-2, changes in biofilm formation were observed in growth rates, production of antimicrobial substances, mobility, secretion of toxins in chemotaxis and colonization with strains in the absence of this protein (Quinones et al., 2009).

Most species of *Campylobacter* have functional LuxS enzymes and are capable of producing AI-2 (Plummer, 2012). However, the presence of nutrients for the production of AI-2 is needed, and these are found in food sources such as milk and juice of chicken meat ("chicken juice"), even in adverse conditions such as oxidative stress and low temperatures (Tazumi et al., 2011; Ligowska et al., 2011; Plummer, 2012).

Treatment and Control

The campylobacteriosis generally is a self-limiting infection that can be treated with fluid therapy, and mostly does not require administration of antibiotics, which are used only with severe infections or septicemia (Alves, 2006; Murray et al., 2009).

In severe cases, the antimicrobial agents of choice are erythromycin, clarithromycin and azithromycin, with best results when the signs are observed in the initial phase and the treatment started before the third day of the symptoms' manifestation (Campderá et al., 2007). Generally these antimicrobials can reduce and eliminate the microorganism in feces.

Children with diarrhea originated by *C. jejuni* demonstrated rapid improvement with early treatment with erythromycin or azithromycin, however, fluoroquinolones to children younger than 12 years is not advisable with risk of growth losses. Clinical experience and studies demonstrated that the treatment with antibiotics is advisable in patients with high fever, bloody stools and diarrhea with more than eight evacuations daily (García; Cravioto, 2007).

Although no clinical efficacy trials have been conducted on animals, it was reported that erythromycin (which is the drug of choice in humans) in doses from 11.1 to 15.5 mg/kg, orally, three times daily for seven days, eliminated the infection in dogs and cats (Holt, 1994). The prognosis is considered good and antibiotics are rapidly effective to stop the elimination of fecal microorganisms.

The resistance of *Campylobacter* to antimicrobials commonly used is a current issue that is under discussion both in the context of veterinary and in human medicine. The occurrence of resistant strains to multiple antibiotics, including the choice for the human treatment limits the therapeutic options in the management of infectious diseases.

According to the CDC (2013) the rates of antibiotic resistance by microorganisms isolated from humans, especially to fluoroquinolones, have risen sharply in the past two decades, and these high rates of resistance are seen today in many regions of the world. When the resistance to fluoroquinolones is proven, azithromycin (macrolide) is generally the next choice of treatment, although resistance to this class of antimicrobials has also already been reported.

Since campylobacteriosis is transmitted by food consumption, the indiscriminate use of these antibiotics in the different stages in chain production of chickens can arrise the spread of resistant strains. Various reports around the world associate infections by *Campylobacter* resistant to fluoroquinolones with the approval of antimicrobial use in poultry chain production (Serichantalergs et al., 2007).

Rastall (2004) investigated alternative antibiotics sources for campylobacteriosis treatment and found that the use of a probiotic (*Lactobacillus acidophilus*) combined with a prebiotic (fructo-oligosaccharides, and lactosucrose) showed good effects on the balance of intestinal microflora, an improvement in infection and immune's recovery. This balance of microflora occurs by competitive exclusion of pathogens after the use of probiotics (Rinkinen, 2003).

The control of human *Campylobacter* infections should begin with actions to reduce infection rates of animal reservoirs of production, and consequently, the harm of their presence in food of animal origin. During the slaughter, sanitary practices should be implemented to prevent cross-contamination, and adequate equipments, facilities and tools sanitization.

In homes and restaurants, enteric campylobacteriosis can be prevented by proper preparation of food, particularly poultry, avoiding consumption of unpasteurized dairy products and implementing measures to prevent contamination of water supplies. Since viable *Campylobacter spp.* is sensitive to heat, the consumption of properly cooked poultry meat seems to be a good measure of control to prevent infection by the bacteria (Allos, 2001), moreover, the prevention of cross-contamination during food preparation (Gonçalves et al., 2012). It is unlikely that the carrier status of *Campylobacter* in animal reservoirs, such as chickens and turkeys will be eliminated. Thus, the risk of infection from these animals still exist (Murray et al., 2009).

The transmission of disease from pet to man is a pathway for the spread of infection. Human cases are associated with recently acquired dogs and cats with diarrhea. The veterinarian should advise the owner of the infected practicing appropriate hygiene measures as an animal: perform a thorough hand washing after contact with animals, promote the proper disposal of contaminated feces, cleaning in place where animals deposit their feces and separate infected animals babies and small children until the cultures after treatment confirm that the infection has cleared (Ettinger, 1992).

Conclusion

Since its recognition as an important zoonotic agent, *Campylobacter* has emerged as the leading bacteria cause of foodborne gastroenteritis in developed countries. Only this finding incites already and demonstrates the need for a broad understanding of the pathogenesis and epidemiology of this microorganism, which can only be achieved with constant and varied studies.

The species of *Campylobacter* have different mechanisms of adaptation and virulence. Knowing the nature of the regulation of these mechanisms allows us to understand their life's cycle, and it is essential to identify the potential hazards of different sources of infection and the ways in which the disease states in humans and animals.

The ability to adhere, to penetrate, invade and cause apoptosis in the human intestinal mucosa represent the main strategies to develop *Campylobacter* infection. Already adaptation strategies that ensure their survival in the environment include genes of tolerance to thermal variations, antimicrobial resistance, oxidative and nutritional stress and the ability to form biofilms. All these intrinsic or acquired mechanisms guarantee the evolutionary success of these microorganisms and disease establishment.

Therefore, studies are essential and constant monitoring through effective epidemiological surveillance systems, including the determination of *Campylobacter* prevalence in animal products throughout the supply chain. Identifying and understanding their virulence characteristics, adaptation and dissemination of genotypes and phenotypes conducted in parallel in strains isolated from human infections, is the appropriate way to identify the sources of infection, the spread of more virulent genotypes and phenotypes, and at the same time create control strategies substantiated for its control.

References

Aarestrup, F. M. (2005).Veterinary drug usage and antimicrobial resistance in bacteria of animal origin. *Basic & Clinical Pharmacology & Toxicology*, *96*, 271-281.

AbuOun, M., Manning, G., Cawthraw, S. A., Ridley, A., Ahmed, I. H., Wassenaar, T. M. & Newell, D. G. (2005). Cytolethal distending toxin (CDT)-negative *Campylobacter jejuni* strains and anti-CDT neutralizing antibodies are induced during human infection but not during colonization in chickens. *Infection and Immunity*, *73*, 3053-3062.

Allos, B. M. (2001). *Campylobacter jejuni* infections: update on emerging issues and trends. *Clinical Infecious Diseases*, *32*, 1201-1206.

Alves, E. Cefar em notícias. Ed 16. São Paulo: Informativo Cefar de Microbiologia - Atualidades científicas - *Campylobacter*; 2006.

Amri, A., Senok, A., Ismaeel, A., Al-Mahmeed, A. & Botta, G. (2007). Multiplex PCR for direct identification of *Campylobacter* spp. in human and chicken stools. *Journal of Medical Microbiology*, *56*, 1350-1355.

Asakura, M., Samosornsuk, W., Taguchi, M., Kobayashi, K., Misawa, N., Kusumoto, M., Nishimura, K., Matsuhisa, A. & Yamasaki, S. (2007). Comparative analysis of citolethal distending toxin (cdt) genes among *Campylobacter jejuni*, *C. coli* and *C. fetus* strains. *Microbial Pathogenesis*, *42*, 174-183.

Axelsson-Olsson, D., Waldenstrom, J., Broman, T., Olsen, B. & Holmberg, M. (2005). Protozoan *Acanthamoeba polyphaga* as a potential reservoir for *Campylobacter jejuni*. *Applied and Environmental Microbiology*, *71*, 987-992.

Bacon, D. J., Alm, R. A., Burr, D. H., Hu, L, Kopecko, D. J., Ewing, C. P., Trust, T. J. & Guerry, P. (2000). Involvement of a plasmid in virulence of *Campylobacter jejuni* 81-176. *Infection and Immunity*, *68*, 4384-4390.

Bandara, H. M. H. N., Lam, O. L. T., Jin, L. J. & Lakshman, S. (2012). Microbial chemical signaling: a current perspective. *Critical Reviews in Microbiology*, *38*, 217-249.

Barker, J., Brown, M. R., Collier, P. J., Farrell, I. & Gilbert, P. (1992). Relationship between *Legionella pneumophila* and *Acanthamoeba polyphaga*: physiological status and susceptibility to chemical inactivation. *Applied and Environmental Microbiology*, *58*, 2420–2425

Bassler, B. L. (1999). How bacteria talk to each other: regulation of gene expression by quorum sensing. *Current Opinion in Microbiology*, *2*, 582-587.

Beales, N. (2004). Adaptation of microorganims to cold temperatures, weak acid preservatives, low pH, and osmotic stress: a review. *Comprehensive Reviews in Food Science and Food Safety*, *3*, 1-20.

Bhavsar, S. & Kapadnis, B. (2007). Virulence factors of *Campylobacter*. *The Internet Journal of Microbiology*, *3*.

Blackwell, G. Regulation of flagellin glycosylation genes in *Campylobacter jejuni*: influence of NssR, the nitrosative stress response regulator. Thesis of doctorate - The University of Birmingham, 278 p., 2010.

Botteldoorn, N., Van Coillie, E., Piessens, V. Rasschaert, G., Debruyne, L., Heyndrickx, M., Herman, L. & Messens, W. (2008). Quantification of *Campylobacter* spp. in chicken carcass rinse by real-time PCR. *Journal of Applied Microbiology*, *105*, 1909-1918.

Brasil, Ministério da Saúde. Protocolo Clínico e Diretrizes Terapêuticas. Síndrome de Guillain-Barré. Portaria SAS/MS n° 497, de 23 de dezembro de 2009.

Campdera, G. A. J., Fernandez, R. R. & Sanchez. M. I. G. (2007). Gastroenteritis por *Salmonella*, *Shigella* y *Campylobacter*.

CDC - Centers for Disease Control and Prevention. (2012). *Campylobacter* investigation Guideline. Kansas Disease Investigation Guidelines.

CDC - Centers For Disease Control and Prevention. (2013). Travelers' Health. In: Mahon, B.E. Chapter 3: Infectious Diseases Related To Travel: Campylobacteriosis.

CFSPH - Centre for Food Security & Public Health. (2005). Animal Disease Factsheets. Available in: http://www.cfsph.iastate.edu. Accessed in: Oct 16 2014.

Chiapparrone, M. L., Morán, P. E., Pasucci, J. A., Echevarría, H. M., Monteavaro, C., Soto, P., Rodríguez, E. & Catena, M. C. (2011). Quantitative analysis of *Campylobacter fetus* venerealis adhesion to bovine reproductive tract cell cultures. *Brazilian Journal of Veterinary Research and Animal Science*, *48*, 73-78.

Corsaro, D., Feroldi, V., Saucedo, G., Ribas, F., Loret, J. F. & Greub, G. (2009). Novel Chlamydiales strains isolated from a water treatment plant. *Environmental Microbiology*, *11*, 188-200.

Crushell, E., Harty, S., Sharif, F. & Bourke, B. (2004). Enteric *Campylobacter*: Purging its Secrets? Pediatric Research Journal [online], 55, 3-12.

Dasti, J. I., Tareen, A. M., Lugert, R., Zautner, A. E. & Gross, U. (2010). *Campylobacter jejuni*: A brief over view on pathogenicity-associated factors and disease-mediating mechanisms. *International Journal of Medical Microbiology, 300*, 205–211.

Davis, M. A. & Conner, D. E. (2007). Survival of *Campylobacter jejuni* on poultry skin and meat at varying temperatures. *Poultry Science, 86*, 765-767.

Dimitraki, P. & Velonakis, E. (2007). The survival of pathogens in frozen food as a health risk. *Archives of Hellenic Medicine, 24*, 432-439.

EFSA - European Food Safety Authority. (2009). The Community Summary Report on Trends and Sources of Zoonoses and Zoonotic Agents in the European Union in 2007. *The EFSA Journal*. Italy, p. 223.

EFSA - European Food Safety Authority. (2010). Analysis of the baseline survey on the prevalence of *Campylobacter* in broiler batches and of *Campylobacter* and *Salmonella* on broiler carcasses in the EU, 2008, *The EFSA Journal*. Italy, 8, n. 3, p. 1503.

Ellis-Iversen, J., Pritchard, G., Wooldridge, M. & Nielen, M. (2009). Risk Factors for *Campylobacter jejuni* and *Campylobacter coli* in young cattle on English and Welsh farms. *Preventive Veterinary Medicine, 88*, 42-48.

Engebrecht, J. & Silverman, M. R. (1984). *Identification of genes and gene products necessary for bacterial bioluminescence. Proceedings of the National Academy of Sciences of the United States of America, 81*, 4154-4158.

Ettinger, S. J. Infecções bacterianas do trato intestinal. In: . Tratado de medicina interna veterinária: molésias do cão e do gato. Tradução de Sônia de Aguiar Gomes do Nascimento e Fernando Gomes do Nascimento. 3. Ed. São Paulo: Manole; 1992, p. 280.

Fàbrega, A., Sánchez-Céspedes, J., Soto, S. & Vila, J. (2008). Quinolone resistance in the food chain. *International Journal of Antimicrobial Agents, 31*, 307-315.

FAO/WHO. (2009). Risk assessment of *Campylobacter* spp. in broiler chickens: Technical Report. Microbiological Risk Assessment Series No. 12. Geneva. 132pp.

Feistel, J. C. Mecanismos de patogenicidade de *Campylobacter* spp. isoladas em alimentos. Seminários Aplicados - Programa de Pós-Graduação em

Ciência Animal da Escola de Veterinária e Zootecnia da Universidade Federal de Goiás, 32p., 2011.

Fernández, H., Villanueva, M.P. & Medina, G. (2012). Endosymbiosis of *Arcobacter butzleri* in *Acanthamoeba castellanii*. Revista Argentina de Microbiología, 44, 133.

Flanagan, R. C., Neal-Mckinney, J. M., Dhillon, A. S., Miller, W. G. & Konkel, M. E. (2009). Examination of *Campylobacter jejuni* putative adhesions leads to the identification of a new protein, designated FlpA, required for chicken colonization. *Infection and Immunity*, 77, 2399-2407. Available in: http://iai.asm.org/cgi/content/abstract/77/6/2399. Accessed in: Aug 28 2014.

Franchin, P. R., Ogliari, P. J. & Batista, C. R. V. (2007). Frequency of thermophilic *Campylobacter* in broiler chickens during industrial processing in a Southern Brazil slaughterhouse. *British Poultry Science*, *48*, 127-132.

García, C. E. & Cravioto, Q. A. (2007). *Campylobacter* y enfermedades asociadas. *Revista de Faculdade de Medicina UNAM*, *50*, 31-35.

Gonçalves, K. O., Yamanaka, E. H. U., Almeida, A. P. I., Chano, L. J. & Ribeiro, A. B. (2012). Pesquisa de *Campylobacter* spp. em carnes de frango comercializados na cidade de Campo Mourão-PR. *Alimentos e Nutrição*, *23*, 211-216.

Greub, G. & Raoult, D. (2004). Microorganisms resistant to free-living amoebae. *Clinical Microbiology Reviews*, *17*, 413-433.

Guerry, P., Alm, R., Szymanski, C. & Trust, T. J. Structure, function, and antigenicity of *Campylobacter* flagella. In: Nachamkin, I. & Blaser, M. J. (ed.), 2nd ed. *Campylobacter*. Washington, D.C.: American Society for Microbiology Press, 2000, 405-421.

Guerry, P. (2007). *Campylobacter* flagella: not just for motility. *Trends in Microbiology*, *15*, 456-461.

Habib, I., Berkvens, D., Zutter, L., Dierick, K., Huffel, X., Speybroeck, N., Geeraerd, A. H. & Uyttendaele, M. (2012). *Campylobacter* contamination in broiler carcasses and correlation with slaughterhouses operational hygiene inspection. *Food Microbiology*, *29*, 105-112.

Han, K., Jang, S. S., Choo, E., Heu, S. & Ryu, S. (2007). Prevalence, genetic diversity and antibiotic resistance patterns of *Campylobacter jejuni* from retail raw chickens in Korea. *International Journal of Food Microbiology*, *114*, 50-59.

Hoffmann, R. & Michel, R. (2001). Distribution of free-living amoebae (FLA) during preparation and supply of drinking water. *International Journal of Hygiene and Environmental Health*, *203*, 215-219.

Holmes, K., Tavender, T. J., Winzer, K., Wells, J. M. & Hardie, K. R. (2009). AI-2 does not function as a quorum sensing molecule in *Campylobacter jejuni* during exponential growth in vitro. *BMC Microbiology*, *9*, 214.

Holt, J. G. (1994). Bergey's Manual of determinative Bacteriology. 9. ed. Baltimore: Williams e Wilkins.

Hu, L. & Kopecko, D. J. (2000). Interactions of *Campylobcater* with eukaryotic cells: gut luminal colonisation and mucosal invasion mechanisms. In: Nachamkin, I. & Blaser, M. J. (ed.), 2nd ed. *Campylobacter*. Washington D.C.: American Society for Microbiology Press, 191-215.

Humphrey, T., O'brien, S. & Madsen, M. (2007). *Campylobacters* as zoonotic pathogens: a food production perspective. *International Journal of Food Microbiology*, *117*, 237–257.

Jang, K. I., Kim, M. G., Ha, S. D., Kim, K. S., Lee, K. H., Chung, D. H., Kim, C. H. & Kim, K. Y. (2007). Morphology and adhesion of *Campylobacter jejuni* to chicken skin under varying conditions. *Journal of Microbiology and Biotechnology*, *17*, 202-206.

Jayaraman, A. & Wood, T. K. (2008). Bacterial quorum sensing: signals, circuits, and implications for biofilms and disease. *Annual Review of Biomedical Engineering*, *10*, 145-167.

Jore, S., Viljugrein, H., Brun, E., Heier, B. T., Borck, B., Ethelberg, S., Hakkinen, M., Kuusi, M., Reiersen, J., Hansson, I., Engvall, E. O., Lofdahl, M., Wagenaar, J. A., Van, P. W., Hofshagen, M. (2010). Trends in *Campylobacter* incidence in broilers and humans in six European countries, 1997-2007. *Preventive Veterinary Medicine*, *93*, 33-41.

Keller, J., Wieland, B., Wittwer, M., Stephan, R. & Perreten, V. (2007). Distribution and genetic variability among *Campylobacter* spp. isolates from different animal species and humans in Switzerland. *Zoonoses Public Health*, *54*, 2-7.

Khanna, M. R., Bhavsar, S. P. & Kapadnis, B. P. (2006). Effect of temperature on growth and chemotactic behaviour of *Campylobacter jejuni*. *Applied Microbiology*, *43*, 84-90.

Khan, N. A. (2006). Acanthamoeba: biology and increasing importance in human health. *FEMS Microbiology Reviews*, *30*, 564-595.

Kilvington, S. & Price, J. (1990). Survival of *Legionella pneumophila* within cysts of *Acanthamoeba polyphaga* following chlorine exposure. *Journal of Applied Bacteriology*, *68*, 519–525.

King, C. H., Shotts, E. B., Wooley, R. E. & Porter, K. G. (1988). Survival of coliforms and bacterial pathogens within protozoa during chlorination. *Applied and Environmental Microbiology*, *54*, 3023-3033.

Konkel, M. E., Kim, B. J., Klena, J. D., Young, C. R. & Ziprin, R. (1998). Characterization of the thermal stress response of *Campylobacter jejuni*. *Infection and Immunity*, *66*, 3666-3672.

Konkel, M. E., Klena, J. D., Rivera-Amill, V., Monteville, M. R., Biswas, D., Raphael, B., Mickelson, J. (2004). Secretion of virulence proteins from *Campylobacter jejuni* is dependent on a functional flagellar export apparatus. *Journal of Bacteriology*, *186*, 3296-3303.

Konkel, M. E., Monteville, M. R., Rivera-Amill, V. & Joens, L. A. (2001). The pathogenesis of *Campylobacter jejuni*-mediated enteritis. *Current Issues in Intestinal Microbiology*, *2*, 55-71.

Korolik, V. & Ketley, J. M. (2005). *Campylobacter* chemotaxis. In: Ketley, J. M. & Konkel, M. E. (ed.), 2nd ed. *Campylobacter*: Molecular and Cellular Biology. Wymondham: Horizon Bioscience UK, 349p.

Krause-Gruszczynska, M., Rohde, M., Hartig, R., Genth, H., Schmidt, G., Keo, T., König, W., Miller, W. G., Konkel, M.E. & Backert, S. (2007). Role of the small Rho GTPases Rac1 and Cdc42 in host cell invasion of *Campylobacter jejuni*. *Cellular Microbiology*, *9*, 2431-2444.

Krause-Gruszczynska, M., Van Alphen, L. B., Oyarzabal, O. A., Alter, T., Hanel, I., Schliephake, A., Konig, W., Van Putten, J. P., Konkel, M. E., Backert, S. (2007). Expression patterns and role of the CadF protein in *Campylobacter jejuni* and *Campylobacter coli*. FEMS Microbiology Letters, 274, 9-16. Available in: http://www.ncbi.nlm.nih.gov/pubmed/17573935. Accessed in: Aug 30 2014.

Kuana, S. L., Santos, L. R., Rodrigues, L. B., Borsoi, A., Moraes, H. L. S., Salle, C. T. P., & Nascimento, V. P. (2008). Occurrence and characterization of *Campylobacter* in the Brazilian production and processing of broilers. *Avian Diseases*, *52*, 680-684.

Kudirkiene, E., Malakauskas, A., Serniene, L. & Malakauskas, M. (2008). Isolation and identification of thermophilic *Campylobacter* spp. by PCR-RFLP in broilers flocks. *Veterinarija Ir Zootechnika*, *42*, 44-47.

Lee, A., Smith, S. C. & Coloe, P. J. (1998). Survival and growth of *Campylobacter jejuni* after artificial inoculation onto chicken skin as a function of temperature and packaging conditions. *Journal of Food Protection*, *61*, 1609-1614.

Levin, R. (2007). *Campylobacter jejuni*: a review of its characteristics, pathogenicity, ecology, distribution, subspecies characterization and molecular methods of detection. *Food Biotechnology*, *21*, 271-347.

Ligowska, M., Cohn, M. T., Stabler, R. A., Wren, B. W. & Brondsted, L. (2011). Effect of chicken meat environment on gene expression of *Campylobacter jejuni* and its relevance to survival in food. *International Journal of Food Microbiology*, *145*, S111-S115.

Malik-Kale, P. Alteration of genetic content and gene expression modulate the pathogenic potential of *Campylobacter jejuni*. Thesis of doctorate - Washington State University - School of Molecular Biosciences, 212 p., 2008.

Malik-Kale, P., Raphael, B. H., Parker, C. T., Joens, L. A., Klena, J. D., Quiñones, B., Keech, A. M. & Konkel, M. E. (2007). Characterization of genetically-matched isolates of *Campylobacter jejuni* reveals mutations in genes involved in flagellar biosynthesis alter the organism's virulence potential. *Applied and Environmental Microbiology*, *73*, 3123-3136.

Marchant, J., Wren, B. & Ketley, J. (2002). Exploiting genome sequence: predictions for mechanisms of *Campylobacter* chemotaxis. *Trends in Microbiology*, *10*, 155-159, 2002.

Matoba, Y., Katsube, Y. & Sugiyama, M. (2002). The crystal structure of prokaryotic phospholipase A2. *The Journal of Biological Chemistry*, *277*, 20059-20069.

Medina, G., Flores-Martin, S., Fonseca, B. B., Otth, C. & Fernández, H. (2014). Mechanisms associated with phagocytosis of *Arcobacter butzleri* by *Acanthamoeba castellanii*. *Parasitology Research*, *113*, 1933-1942.

Melo, R. T. (2012). Fatores de patogenicidade e potencial risco à saúde em *Campylobacter* spp. isolados de carcaças de frangos. Dissertação de Mestrado em Ciência Animal – Faculdade de Medicina Veterinária - Universidade Federal de Uberlândia, 133 p.

Mihaljevic, R. R., Sikic, M., Klancnik, A., Brumini, G., Mozina, S. S. & Abram, M. (2007). Environmental stress factors affecting survival and virulence of *Campylobacter jejuni*. *Microbial Pathogenesis*, *43*, 120-125.

Miller, C. E., Williams, P. H. & Ketley, J. M. (2009). Pumping iron: mechanisms for iron uptake by *Campylobacter*. *Microbiology*, *155*, 3157-3165.

Monteville, M. R., Yoon, J. E. & Konkel, M. E. (2003). Maximal adherence and invasion of INT 407 cells by *Campylobacter jejuni* requires the *CadF* outer membrane protein and microfilament reorganization. *Microbiology*, 149, 153-165.

Moore, J. E., Barton, M. D., Blair, I. S., Corcoran, D., Dooley, J. S. G., Fanning, S., Kempf, I., Lastovica, A. J., Lowery, C. J., Matsuda, M., Mcdowell, D. A., Mcmahon, A., Millar, B. C., Rao, J. R., Rooney, P. J., Seal, B. S., Snelling, W. J. & Tolba, O. (2006). The epidemiology of antibiotic resistance in *Campylobacter. Microbes and Infection*, *8*, 1955-1966.

Moore, J. E., Corcoran, D., Dooley, J. S. G., Fanning, S., Lucey, B., Matsudda, M., Mcdowell, D. A., Mégraud, F., Millar, B. C., O'mahony, R., O'riordan, L., O'rourke, M., Rao, J. R., Rooney, P. J., Ssais, A. & Whyte, P. (2005). *Campylobacter. Veterinary Researche*, *36*, 351-382.

Muraoka, W. T. & Zhang, Q. (2011). Phenotypic and genotypic evidence for L-fucose utilization by *Campylobacter jejuni. Journal of Bacteriology*, *193*, 1065-1075.

Murray, P. R., Baron, E. J., Jorgensen, J. H., Landry, M. L. & Pfaller, M. A. (2007). Manual of Clinical Microbiology, 9 ed., Washington, D.C.: American Society for Microbiology Press.

Murray, P. R., Rosenthal, K. S. & Pfaller, M. A. (2009). *Campylobacter* e *Helicobacter*. In:_____. Microbiologia médica. 6 ed. Rio de Janeiro: Elsevier, 948 p.

Olofsson, J., Axelsson-Olsson, D., Brudin. L, Olsen. B, Ellström. P. (2013). *Campylobacter jejuni* actively invades the amoeba *Acanthamoeba polyphaga* and survives within non digestive vacuoles. *PLOS One*, *8*, e78873.

Parkhill, J., Wren, B. W., Mungall, K., Ketley, J. M., Churcher, C., Basham, D., Chillingworth, T., Davies, R. M., Feltwell, T., Holroyd, S., Jagels, K., Karlyshev, A. V., Moule, S., Pallen, M. J., Penn, C. W., Quail, M. A., Rajandream, M. A., Rutherford, K. M., Van Vliet, A. H., Whitehead, S. & Barrell, B. G. (2000). The genome sequence of the food-borne pathogen *Campylobacter jejuni* reveals hypervariable sequences. *Nature*, *403*, 665- 668.

Parveen, N., & Cornell, K. A. (2011). Methylthioadenosine/S-adenosylhomocysteine nucleosidase, a critical enzyme for bacterial metabolism. *Molecular Microbiology*, *79*, 7-20.

Pope, J. E., Krizova, A., Garg, A. X., Thiessen-Philbrook, H. & Ouimet, J. M. (2007). *Campylobacter* reactive arthritis: a systematic review. *Seminars in Arthritis and Rheumatism*, *37*, 48-55.

Quinones, B., Miller, W. G., Bates, A. H. & Mandrell, R. E. (2009). Autoinducer-2 production in *Campylobacter jejuni* contributes to chicken colonization. *Applied and Environmental Microbiology*, *75*, 281-285.

Rabinstein, A. A. (2007). Guillain-Barré Syndrome. *The Open General and Internal Medicine Journal*, *1*, 13–22.

Rajan, R., Zhu, J., Hu, X., Pei, D. & Bell, C. E. (2005). Crystal structure of S-ribosylhomocysteinase (LuxS) in complex with a catalytic 2-ketone intermediate. *Biochemistry*, *44*, 3745-3753.

Rastall, R. A. (2004). Bacteria in the gut: friends and foes and how to alter the balance. *The Journal of Nutrition*, *134*, 2022-2026.

Reid, A. N., Pandey, R., Palyada, K., Naikare, H. & Stintzi, A. (2008). Identification of *Campylobacter jejuni* genes involved in the response to acidic pH and stomach transit. *Applied and Environmental Microbiology*, *74*, 1583-1597.

Ridley, A. M., Allen, V. M., Sharma, M., Harris, J. A. & Newell, D. G. (2008). Real-time PCR approach for detection of environmental sources of *Campylobacter* strains colonizing broiler flocks. *Applied and Environmental Microbiology*, *74*, 2492-2504.

Rinkinen, M., Jalava, K., Westermarck, E., Salminen, S. & Ouwehand, A. C. (2003). Interaction between probiotic lactic acid bacteria and canine enteric pathogens: a risk factor for intestinal *Enterococcus faecium* colonization? *Veterinary Microbiology*, *92*, 111-119.

Rivera-Amill, V., Kim, B. J., Seshu, J. & Konkel, M. E. (2001). Secretion of the virulence associated *Campylobacter* invasion antigens from *Campylobacter jejuni* requires a stimulatory signal. *Journal of Infectious Diseases*, *183*, 1607-1616.

Sallam, K. I. (2007). Prevalence of *Campylobacter* in chicken and chicken by-products retailed in Sapporo area, Hokkaido, Japan. *Food Control*, *18*, 1113-1120.

Sampers, I., Habib, I., Berkvens, D., Dumoulin, A., Zutter, L. D. & Uyttendaele, M. (2009). Processing practices contributing to *Campylobacter* contamination in Belgian chicken meat preparations. *International Journal of Food Microbiology*, *128*, 297-303.

Schmidt-Ott, R., Pohl, S., Burghard, S., Weig, M. & Gross, U. (2005). Identification and characterization of a major subgroup of conjugative *Campylobacter jejuni* plasmids. *Journal of Infection*, *50*, 12-21.

Scientific Status Summary. Bacteria associated whit foodborne diseases. Institute of Food Technologistis, Chicago, 1-25, 2004.

Serichantalergs, O., Dalsgaard, A., Bodhidatta, L., Krasaesub, S., Pitarangsi, C., Srijan, A. & Mason, C. J. (2007). Emerging fluoroquinolone and macrolide resistance of *Campylobacter jejuni* and *Campylobacter coli* isolates and their serotypes in Thai children from 1991 to 2000. *Epidemiology and Infection*, *135*, 1299-1306.

Silva, J., Leite, D., Fernandes, M., Mena, C., Gibbs, P. A. & Teixeira, P. (2011). *Campylobacter* spp. as a foodborne pathogen: a review. *Frontiers in Microbiology*, *2*, 1-12.

Silva, N., Junqueira, V. C. A., Silveira, N. F. A., Taniwaki, M. H., Santos, R. F. S. & Gomes, R. A. R. (2007). Manual de métodos de análise microbiológica de alimentos. 3 ed., São Paulo: Livraria Varela.

Smith, J. L. & Bayles, D. O. (2006). The contribution of cytolethal distending toxin to bacterial pathogenesis. *Critical Reviews in Microbiology*, 32, 227-248. Available in: http://www.ncbi.nlm.nih.gov/pubmed/17123907. Accessed in: Aug 18 2014.

Snelling, W. J., Matsuda, M., Moore, J. E. & Dooley, J. S. (2005). *Campylobacter jejuni*. *Letters in Applied Microbiology*, *41*, 297-302.

Snelling, W. J., McKenna, J. P., Lecky, D. M. & Dooley, J. S. (2005). Survival of *Campylobacter jejuni* in waterborne Protozoa. *Applied and Environmental Microbiology*, *71*, 5560-5571.

Stintzi, A. (2003). Gene expression profile of *Campylobacter jejuni* in response to growth temperature variation. *Journal of Bacteriology*, *185*, 2009-2016.

Stintzi A. & Whitworth L. (2003). Investigation of the *Campylobacter jejuni* cold-shock response by global transcript. *Genome Letters*, *2*, 18-27.

Tazumi, A., Negoro, M., Tomiyama, Y., Misawa, N., Itoh, K., Moore, J. E., Millar, B. C., & Matsuda, M. (2011).Uneven distribution of the luxS gene within the genus *Campylobacter*. *British Journal of Biomedical Science*, *68*, 19-22.

Thomas, V., Loret, J. F., Jousset, M. & Greub, G. (2008). Biodiversity of amoebae and amoebae resisting bacteria in a drinking water treatment plant. *Environmental Microbiology*, *10*, 2728–2745.

Vucic, S., Kiernan, M. C. & Cornblath, D. R. (2009). Guillain-Barré syndrome: an update. *Journal of Clinical Neuroscience*, *16*, 733-741.

Wassenaar, T. M., Van Der Zeijst, B. A., Ayling, R. & Newell, D. G. (1993). Colonization of chicks by motility mutants of *Campylobacter jejuni* demonstrates the importance of flagellin A expression. *Journal of General Microbiology*, *139*, 1171-1175.

WHO - World Health Organization. Water-related diseases. 2011. Available in: http://www.who.int/water_sanitation_health/diseases/campylobacteriosis/en/. Accessed in: Aug 23 2014.

Xavier, K. B. & Bassler, B. L. (2005). Interference with AI-2-mediated bacterial cell-cell communication. *Nature*, *437*, 750-753.

Xu, H., Lee, H. Y. & Ahn, J. (2008). Cross-protective effect of acid-adapted *Salmonella enterica* on resistance to lethal acid and cold stress conditions. *Letters in Applied Microbiology*, *47*, 290-297.

Zilbauer, M., Dorrell, N., Wren, B. W. & Bajaj-Elliott, M. (2008). *Campylobacter jejuni*-mediated disease pathogenesis: an update. *Transactions of the Royal Society of Tropical Medicine and Hygiene*, *102*, 123-129.

Ziprin, R. L., Young, C. R., Byrd, J. A., Stanker, L. H., Hume, M. E., Gray, S. A., Kim, B. J. & Konkel, M. E. (2001). Role of *Campylobacter jejuni* potential virulence genes in cecal colonization. *Avian Diseases*, *45*, 549-557.

In: Campylobacter Infections
Editor: Brittany A. Bertucci
ISBN: 978-1-63463-858-6

Chapter 5

Campylobacter Infections: Epidemiology, Clinical Management and Prevention. Our Twenty Five-Year Experience in Greece

A. Ioannidis[1,3], E. Magiorkinis[2*], V. Ioannidou[3], S. Perlorentzou[2] and S. Chatzipanagiotou[3]

[1]Department of Nursing, Faculty of Human Movement and Quality of Life Sciences, University of Peloponnese, Greece
[2]Department of Microbiology, Metaxas Memorial Anticancer Hospital, Pireas, Greece
[3]Department of Biopathology and Clinical Microbiology, Aeginition Hospital, Athens Medical School, Greece

Abstract

Campylobacteriosis caused principally by *Campylobacter jejuni* and *Campylobacter coli*, is among the main causes of bacterial gastroenteritis

* Corresponding author: Emmanouil Magiorkinis, MD, PhD, BSc, Georgiou Papandreou 94, 18900 Salamina, Greece, e-mail: emmanouil.magiorkinis@gmail.com; Tel: +30-210-4677549

worldwide. In developing countries, campylobacteriosis is primarily a disease that occurs during infancy, because of high levels of early exposure and acquired immunity, but in industrialized countries, the epidemiology is characterized by sporadic infection throughout the population at all ages. The consumption of undercooked poultry, unpasteurized milk, improperly treated surface water and traveling abroad are the main sources of human campylobacter infection. Most infections are self-limiting, but antibiotic treatment may be required in cases of prolonged or severe illness and for vulnerable individuals, such as the very young or the very old. An increase in rates of resistance to fluoroquinolones in campylobacter stains from humans has been found associated with the approval of the use of fluoroquinolones (enrofloxacin) in veterinary medicine. Although there is no systematic surveillance and notification of Campylobacter infections in Greece, by retrieving data from various sources from general hospitals, *Campylobacter jejuni* is either the first or the second most common bacterial enteric pathogen (the other one being *Salmonella* ssp.) in our country. The last two decades several epidemiological studies that took place have delineated the epidemiology of Campylobacter in Greece. Serotyping studies have revealed that serotype HS:2 is the most predominant,whereas serotype HS:19 which is link to Guillain-Barré Syndrome (GBS), has also detected. Because of typing systems for Campylobacter epidemiologic studies vary in complexity and abilities to discriminate among strains versatile molecular surveys of characterization of Campylobacter strains based on *flaA* typing through RFLP led to the characterization of 39 differrent *flaA* types (*flaA*1-39 GR), whereas based on PFGE typing, a total of 43 different PFGE types were identified. MLST typing in conjunction with phylogenetic analysis revealed a total of 41 different MLST- sequence types of which 12 were unique in Greece. The studies also demonstrated that *racR* was the gene with the highest prevalence in our strain database. Besides, the resistance to fluoroquinolones in greek strains was not connected with the transferable gene *qnr*A. In conclusion, the Campylobacter infections in Greece, a) there are no notifications about small or large outbreaks, only sporadic cases have been hitherto reported, b) there is no clonality of the isolated strains on molecular level, c) commercially available foods seem not to be transmission sources and d) resistance rates to various antimicrobials agents vary, with those to fluoroquinolones remaining high. The burden of acute disease caused by campylobacter is important and underscores the need to develop effective surveillance systems in order to prevent human illness throughout each link in the food chain.

Introduction

Campylobacter infections have been recognized as an important agent of human morbidity during the last 30 years, especially during the 70's, although there have been significant data since 1947 [1]. *Campylobacter* was initially isolated in 1906 from aborting sheep in the UK by McFadyen and Stockman in 1913 [2]. The clinical symptoms of campylobacteriosis were described much earlier by Theodor Escherich in 1886 in infants [3]. The clinical entity was named as *cholera infantum* or *summer complaint.* The bacteria were characterized as vibrios and were classified as a separate genus with *Vibrio fetus* in 1919 by Smith and Taylor in US [1].The microorganism known today as *Campylobacter jejuni* was identified in 1931 by Jones *et al.* [4] as the causative agent of winter dysentery in cattle. In 1957, King described microaerobic, motile curved rods isolated from the blood of children with acute dysentery, which he characterized as vibrios [5]. In 1963, genetic analysis showed that this new species could not ferment carbohydrates and had a different G+C percentage from other *Vibrio spp.,* and, therefore, was classified as a different genus, named because of their shape *Campylobacter spp.* [2]. In 1977, Skirrow introduced a simple culture method for *Campylobacter* from fecal samples [6]. This method and the development of selective culture media allowed the isolation of this pathogen in diagnostic microbiological laboratories. It was not until the 1970s when *C. jejuni* and *C. coli* were associated with acute enteritis in humans. Other species such as *C. upsaliensis* and *C. lari* have been described as causative agents of acute diarrhea mainly in children in developing countries. *C. fetus* is ~~a~~ the main cause for abortion in sheep, whereas it is a rare cause of fetal infection and abortion in humans and, occasionally, of bacteremia in patients with severe immune deficiency. Other medically important species include *C. concisus* and *C. rectus*, which have been linked with periodental disease.

2. Epidemiology-Clinical Significance

Campylobacter species has been recognized as an emerging human and animal foodborne pathogen. The common routes of infection in humans are fecal-oral, through the consumption of contaminated milk [7, 8], water [9] and undercooked meat, especially poultry [119]. Besides enteritis, in cases of septic arthritis, meningitis and proctocolitis reference has been made to C.

jejuni as the cause [10]]. An association between campylobacteriosis and Guillain-Barré syndrome (GBS) has also been proposed, although the risk of developing GBS is generally small (<1 case of GBS/1,000 infections) [11-18]. As Campylobacter spp. have a world-wide distribution, many sporadic cases are being documented. In those cases it is very difficult to discover the source of infection. [19]. More than 1% of the total population is infected by Campylobacter in developed countries (Europe and the US).

C. coli is the second most important pathogen from the Campylobacter genus; it accounts for 5-10% of campylobacterioses in humans [20]. C. consisus is able to grow anaerobically and has been isolated from human gingival crevices; it has been associated with gastrointestinal disease especially in immunocompromised patients [21]. C. fetus is a rare human pathogen affecting specific patient groups, such as patients with chronic renal, hepatic or neoplastic disease and immunocompromised patients [22, 23]. Other species that have been sporadically associated with human infections include C. hyointestinalis [24, 25], C. jejuni subsp. doylei, C. lari [26, 27], C. mucosalis [28, 29], C. upsaliensis [30-34], C. gracilis [35], C. rectus [36, 37] (Figure 1). Because the infection is usually self-limiting, the true population incidence is estimated to be 8 to 30 times higher than confirmed cases, depending on the country.

3. Bacteriology

Campylobacters are small, curved, S-shaped or spiral gram-negative rods with a single polar flagellum at one or both ends, giving them an exceptional motility, darting motility (0.5-5 μm long and wide 0.2-0.8 μm) [23]. Movement is achieved by a unipolar flagellum. 16S rRNA sequence analysis of microaerobic gram-negative bacteria has shown that *Campylobacter* spp. along with other genera (*Arcobacter, Helicobacter, Wolinella* and *Flexispira*) belong to the same rRNA superfamily (rRNA superfamily VI) (Figure 1) [38, 39]; Campylobacters belong to group I. Till now, more than 20 different species have been characterized within *Campylobacter* genus [40]. Some of them are pathogens for humans and animals and have been isolated from the genital and gastrointestinal tract (Table 1).

The most important pathogens for humans and animals are *C. jejuni* and *C. coli* [2, 19].

They are characterized as microaerobic, since low oxygen concentration is necessary for their growth and they are unusually susceptible to normal oxygen concentration and to superoxides. *C. coli* and especially *C. jejuni* grow best at 37-42°C; for that reason they are both referred to as 'thermophilic campylobacters'. Under adverse conditions, they undergo coccal transformation. *Campylobacters* utilize amino acids and intermediates from the citric acid cycle as sources of energy, but not carbohydrates. Biochemically they are inactive in many conventional biochemical tests such as metabolism of sugars; they do not ferment or oxidize carbohydrates [23]. *C. jejuni* is unable to hydrolyze gelatin, starch, casein, tyrosine but it can effectively hydrolyze hippuric acid. Hippuric acid hydrolysis along with other phenotypic characteristics are used for the laboratory identification in clinical practice [41].

Table 1. *Campylobacter* spp. that have been isolated from humans and animals, whereas C. *avium*, *C. canadensis*, *C. cuniculorum*, *C. subantarcticus*, *C. troglodytis*, *C. volucris*, '*Campylobacter* sp. Dolphin DP', and '*Campylobacter* sp. Prairie Dog')* have been isolated only from animals (until July 2011)

Campylobacter ssp		
C. coli	C. insulaenigrae	C. avium*
C. concisus	C. jejuni subsp. jejuni C. jejuni subsp. doylei	C. canadensis*
C. curvus	C. lanienae	C. cuniculorum*
C. faecalis	C. lari	C. subantarcticus*
C. fetus subsp. fetus	C. mucosalis	C. troglodytis*
C. fetus subsp. venerealis	C. peloridis	C. volucris*
C. gracilis	C. rectus	Campylobacter sp. Dolphin DP*
C. hominis	C. showae	Campylobacter sp. Prairie Dog*
C. helveticus	C. sputorum	
C. hyointestinalis	C. upsaliensis	
C. hyoilei	C. ureolyticus	

All *Campylobacter* spp. are oxidase positive except from *C. gracilis*, whereas they do not produce lipase or lecithinase. Classification of *Campylobacter* spp. was difficult before the introduction of PCR methods since their ability to take up naked DNA led to genetic diversification which could not be detected by conventional techniques. A serotyping system has been developed based on the major antigen (capsular polysaccharide).

4. Laboratory Diagnosis

C. jejuni and *C.coli* continue to be the most common *Campylobacter* species associated with diarrheal illness in humans worldwide. Initially a wet mount of very fresh stool sample (<30 min old) is used to detect motile campylobacters as darting across the field in a zigzag fashion. Fecal white blood cells may be present during *Campylobacter* infection, however the absence of fecal leukocytes does not rule out the diagnosis. Most Campylobacters require a microaerobic environment of 5% O_2 85 % N_2 and 10% CO_2 for optimal growth at 42° C. For detection of species other than *C .jejuni* and *C. coli*, a desired incubation of a second plate at 35 to 37° C is required. A number of selective media are recommended for isolating *C.jejuni* and *C. coli,* such as blood free charcoal-cefoperazone-desoxycholate agar (CCDA) or blood containing media, two of which are Campy CVA medium and Skirrow medium. In general, *Campylobacter* spp. produce gray, flat and irregular spreading along the streak (particularly on freshly prepared media) colonies. A Gram stain examination of the colony reveals characteristic gram-negative, curved to S-shaped rods. *C. jejuni* is easy to identify phenotypically; strains isolated on selective media that grow at 42° C, under microaerobic conditions are oxidase positive, show characteristic microscopic morphology, and give a positive result with hippurate hydrolysis should be reported as *C.jejuni* subsp. *jejuni*

5. Clinical Management and Treatment

The rehydration and maintenance of electrolyte balance is the cornerstone of treatment for *Campylobacter* enteritis (Table 2). Most infections are self-limiting, and do not require antibiotics at all. Nevertheless, there are specific clinical cases in which antibiotics should be used. These include high fevers, bloody diarrhea, prolonged illness (symptoms that last > 1 week from the time of diagnosis), patients with bloodstream infections, pregnancy, infection with HIV and immunocompromised patients. The drugs of choice for treatment are a macrolide (e.g., erythromycin) or fluoroquinolones [42].

However, since 1990, a rapidly increasing proportion of *Campylobacter* strains have been found to be fluoroquinolones-resistant [43]. The main reason for the development of resistance is the reckless use of fluoroquinolones (enrofloxacin, sarafloxacin) in veterinary medicine, which results in the selection of quinolone resistant strains [44]. Erythromycin is returning as the optimal drug for treatment of *Campylobacter* infections, although occasional resistance is also reported with this agent. Nevertheless, the rate of resistance of *Campylobacter* to erythromycin remains quite low [45]. In addition, unlike the fluoroquinolones, erythromycin may be administered safely to children and pregnant women. The newer macrolides, azithromycin and claritromycin, are also effective, but they are more expensive than erythromycin. Given that fluoroquinolone resistance is present in a significant proportion of *Campylobacter* strains, susceptibility testing should be performed in clinical practice.

Table 2. Myths and truths about *Campylobacter*

Myths	Truths
Campylobacter infections are always limited to a mild gastroenteritis.	Most of *Campylobacter* infections are mild and self-limited. However, in vulnerable populations, such as newborns, children, old people, immunosuppressed and immunocompromised individuals, the infection can become very severe with various complications like colitis, appendicitis, toxic megacolon, intestinal hemorrhage, hepatitis, cholecystitis, pancreatitis, peritonitis, myocarditis, nephritis and splenic rupture.
People belonging to the closest family circle of an individual with diagnosed *Campylobacter* infection are designated as "high risk" persons for the acquisition of the infection.	The transmission risk of *Campylobacter* in people close to the patient is theoretical. Practically there are no reports about human to human transmission. This can be explained by the fact that *Campylobacter* cannot survive in ambient conditions, as well as by its high susceptibility to disinfectants and antiseptics. Simple hygienic measures effectively eliminate the risk of transmission.

Table 2. (Continued)

Myths	Truths
The close environment of a patient with *Campylobacter* infection must be carefully disinfected, because the pathogen is very resistant to unfavorable environmental conditions.	*Campylobacter* is very susceptible to ambient conditions and is rapidly destroyed, particularly if the surrounding area is cleaned and disinfected.
The postinfectious immunopathologic syndrome Guillain-Barré (peripheral demyelinating neuropathy) associated with a preceding *Campylobacter* infection, is a mild neurologic disorder with a very good prognosis.	The postinfectious immunopathologic syndrome Guillain-Barré (peripheral demyelinating neuropathy) associated with a preceding *Campylobacter* infection, compared to the one caused by other pathogens, is the most severe and the most commonly linked with irreversible complications.
Meat products, which must be consumed after cooking, derived from potentially infected crops with *Campylobacter* must be withdrawn as inappropriate.	The well cooked meat, especially poultry meat is absolutely safe with respect to *Campylobacter*. However, in case a crop is found positive for *Campylobacter*, the crop must be withdrawn for public health security reasons. As the controls are based on random sampling, if an infected crop "slips through", cooking sufficiently eliminates effectively *Campylobacter* transmission.
The uncontrolled and unjustified therapeutic use of antibiotics has triggered the selection of resistant *Campylobacter* strains to many antimicrobial groups.	The reckless use of antimicrobials in livestock and poultry farming is the main cause for the selection and spread of *Campylobacter* antimicrobial resistant strains worldwide in contrast to what happens with other bacterial pathogens. In most *Campylobacter* infections in adults no antimicrobials are administered, while in children quinolones are contraindicated (an antimicrobial group with increasing resistance rates with respect to *Campylobacter*).

5. Campylobacteriosis in Greece

Although there is no systematic surveillance and notification of *Campylobacter* infections in Greece, by retrieving data from various sources from general hospitals, *Campylobacter jejuni* is either the first or the second most common bacterial enteric pathogen (the other one being Salmonella) in our country. In the present review, our twenty-five – year experience will be presented in brief, gained by studies on *Campylobacter* in Greece.

In the early 90's resistance of *Campylobacter* to fluoroquinolones, an alternative drug for treating erythromycin resistant cases was reported. In 1993 we reported a study regarding strains isolated from 31 infected children and we found 32.2% resistance rates to nalidixic acid, ciprofloxacin, norfloxacin and ofloxacin. As this group of antimicrobials was not used for the treatment of children, it was assumed that those strains might be selected through the use of quinolones in veterinary medicine [45].

In a comparative epidemiological study including 129 strains collected in two time periods, 1987-1988 (group A) and 1998-2000 (group B), susceptibility patterns differed significantly between the two groups with respect to quinolones, with an increase in the percentage of resistant strains in group B (30.6% versus 0% in group A), whereas erythromycin, ampicillin and co-amoxiclav remained effective in both groups [46].

In 2003, the heat stable-serotyping of *Campylobacter* (Penner method) was published. When this method was performed for the first time in Greece, it revealed a variety of serotypes. Serotype HS:2 was predominant, followed by the HS:4 complex and HS:1,44 [47]. Many clinically important Guillain-Barré Syndrome (GBS) associated serotypes, like HS:19 were identified [48].

In 2003 we reported the first diagnosed *C. jejuni*-associated GBS case reported from Greece in a child with previous serotype HS19 infection, with positive nerve ganglioside antibodies and HLA-B35 and HLA-DR8 antigens, which have been found to be associated with previous *C. jejuni* infection in GBS patients. In order to examine the possible involvement of cytokines in GBS, the concentrations of three pro-inflammatory cytokines (interleukin (IL)-2sRa, IL-6 and interferon (IFN)-gamma) and one anti-inflammatory cytokine (IL-10) were measured in peripheral blood mononuclear cells after induction with different *C. jejuni* serotypes. No differences were found for IL-6, IFN-gamma and IL-10, but the non-sialylated serotype HS:3 was associated with decreased production of IL-2sRa.These results raised the possibility that absence of sialylation might be associated with the inability to induce inflammatory factors such as cytokines [49].

Resistance of *C. jejuni* to fluoroquinolones is mainly due to chromosomal mutations in the genes that encode the gyrA and parC subunits of DNA gyrase and topoisomerase IV, respectively. In many gram-negative bacteria, low-level quinolone resistance was found to be due to the protective action on DNA gyrase of QnrA, a 218 amino acid protein of the pentapeptide repeat family. The respective gene, termed *qnrA* was found to be on a transferable 180 kb multiresistance plasmid (pMG252), discovered in a clinical isolate of *Klebsiella pneumoniae*. This gene was absent in all *Campylobacter* isolates of our strain collection [50].

Exploring the presence of four virulence genes (*racR, wlaN, cgtB, virB11*) chosen on the basis of their variation in prevalence in 356 *C. jejuni* clinical strains, the gene with the highest prevalence was *racR* (87.08%). *VirB* was present in only 1.69% of the *C. jejuni* strains, and *wlaN* and *cgtB* were detected in 16.01% and 24.44%, respectively. Five strains associated with Guillain-Barré syndrome and Miller-Fischer syndrome out of the total of 356 (1.40%) were positive for *cgtB*. These results supported that *racR* may encode factors necessary for bacterial pathogenicity in humans, while the roles of the other three genes remain ambiguous [51].

As *Campylobacter* serotyping, yielding many non-typable strains, is of clinical importance, a versatile molecular characterization of *Campylobacter* strains was planned, using highly discriminatory molecular methods, in order to establish data of epidemiological and clinical relevance.

The first method referred to flagellin subunit A gene (*flaA*) typing of *Campylobacter*, through restriction fragment length polymorphism (RFLP), which has been recognized by several groups as a relatively simple and quick genotyping method. A total of 207 *C. jejuni* clinical isolates of known serotype were investigated, collected from 5 general hospitals of the area of Attica, during the period 2000-2003. Thirty nine different *flaA* types, designated as *flaA* 1 GR to *flaA* 39 GR (GR:Greece) were found. There was no significant association of certain genotypes with certain serotypes. However, *flaA* typing showed a remarkable discriminatory ability inside the non-serotypable (NT) group [52].

In a later study including 192 *C. jejuni* isolated in the period 2004-2007, *flaA* typing was investigated with respect to the antimicrobial resistance patterns. A statistically significant correlation between certain *flaA* genotypes (*flaA* 17 Greece [GR], *flaA* 19 GR and *flaA* 39 GR) and resistance to some antimicrobial agents (ampicillin, amoxicillin/clavulanic acid [co-amoxiclav], erythromycin, nalidixic acid, and ciprofloxacin) were detected [53].

Further characterization was performed using analysis by pulsed-field gel electrophoresis (PFGE) after SmaI digestion. A total of 93 *C. jejuni* clinical isolates of known flagellin subunit A (*flaA*) genotype, serotype, and antimicrobial susceptibility pattern, collected from a general hospital in the Attica region of Greece, between the years 2000 and 2003 were included. Forty-three different PFGE types, designated as *C. jejuni* (C. j.) 1 Greece (GR) to C. j. 43 GR, were identified. There was no statistically significant association of PFGE type with *flaA* genotype, serotype, or antimicrobial susceptibility pattern [54].

In 2013, we published data with respect to the molecular epidemiology of *C. jejuni* and *C. coli* clinical strains using the multilocus sequence typing method (MLST) [55]. The MLST genotypes were compared with those gained by other typing methods (HS-typing, PFGE and FlaA typing) and were also phylogenetically analyzed, in order to disclose genetic relationships.

Among 68 *C. jejuni* strains, 41 different MLST-Sequence Types (MLST-STs) were found. Fifty six strains or 34 MLST-STs could be sorted into 15 different MLST-Sequence Type Complexes (MLST-STCs), while twelve strains or seven MLST-STs did not match any of the MLST-STCs of the database. Twenty *C. coli* strains belonged to 14 different MLST-STs. Eleven MLST-STs were classified in the same MLST-STC (828), and three were unclassifiable. There was no significant association between the MLST-STs and the results of the other typing methods. Phylogenetic analysis revealed that some strains, classified to the species of *C. jejuni*, formed a separate, phylogenetically distinct group. In eight strains some alleles belonging to the taxonomic cluster of *C. jejuni*, were also detected in *C. coli* and vice versa, a phenomenon caused by the genetic mosaic encountered inside the genus *Campylobacter*. The MLST-ST determination proved to be a very useful tool for the typing as well as the identification of *Campylobacter* on the species level [55].

Our most recent investigation on *Campylobacter* antimicrobial resistance published in 2007, studied a total of 170 *Campylobacter* jejuni strains isolated from the stool of children, collected during a two-year period (2004-2005) [56]. From the 170 strains 30% were resistant to ciprofloxacin (MIC > or = 4 μg/ml), 55% to tetracycline (MIC > 8 μg/ml), 13% to clindamycin (MIC > or = 8 μg/ml), 4% to ampicillin (MIC > 16 μg/ml), 6% to erythromycin (MIC > or = 8 μg/ml), 4% to coamoxiclav (MIC > or = 16/8 microg/ml) and 0% to gentamicin.

Compared to previous reports from Greece, the antimicrobial resistance rates to erythromycin, ampicillin and coamoxiclav remained low, while they were still high for tetracycline and ciprofloxacin. Considering similar reports from many other countries and the high incidence of *Campylobacter* gastroenteritis worldwide, the value of ciprofloxacin as a first choice drug in the empiric treatment of the infection becomes questionable.

In 2012, we reported results regarding the isolation, identification, and antimicrobial resistance of *Campylobacter* spp. from poultry and raw meat from slaughterhouses. During the period from August 2005 to November 2008, a total of 1080 samples were collected. Sixteen *Campylobacter* strains were isolated, none of the strains was identified as *C. jejuni*, based on 16S rRNA species specific gene amplification by PCR. All the strains were susceptible to ciprofloxacin, amoxicillin-clavulanic acid, and gentamicin. Thirteen out of 14 *C. coli* were resistant to erythromycin and all *C. coli* strains were resistant to ampicillin [57].

In 2001, one of the authors represented Greece in a feasibility study pointing to an effort to establish a European network on human *Campylobacter* infections [58]. Two surveys had been conducted on behalf of the *Campylobacter* Working Group. The first survey, conducted in 18 countries, collected information about diagnostic methods used for surveillance purposes, while the second one, conducted among 10 European countries, gathered data on diagnostic methods and procedures in primary laboratories. Seventeen of the 18 countries had a surveillance system for *Campylobacter* infections and 13, a national reference laboratory. The case definition used for the surveillance in all these countries included laboratory confirmation. No commonly applicable subtyping methods were applied. Concerning primary laboratories dealing with *Campylobacter* infections, only a few of them reported directly to the national level, and antimicrobial susceptibility testing was performed by about half of the laboratories. Although the surveys indicated that a basic infrastructure for a wide European *Campylobacter* surveillance existed, the project was not further materialized, in terms of putting into practice, due to unknown reasons.

Regarding *Campylobacter* infections among the Greek population the following conclusion could be drawn: a) there are no notifications about small or large outbreaks, only sporadic cases have been hitherto reported, b) there is no clonality of the isolated strains on molecular level, c) commercially available foods seem not to be transmission sources and d) resistance rates to the various antimicrobials vary, with those to quinolones remaining high.

Although *Campylobacter* is a very common enteric pathogen in Greece, the lack of small or large outbreaks might be due to the Greek dietary habits avoiding uncooked or undercooked meat products in general.

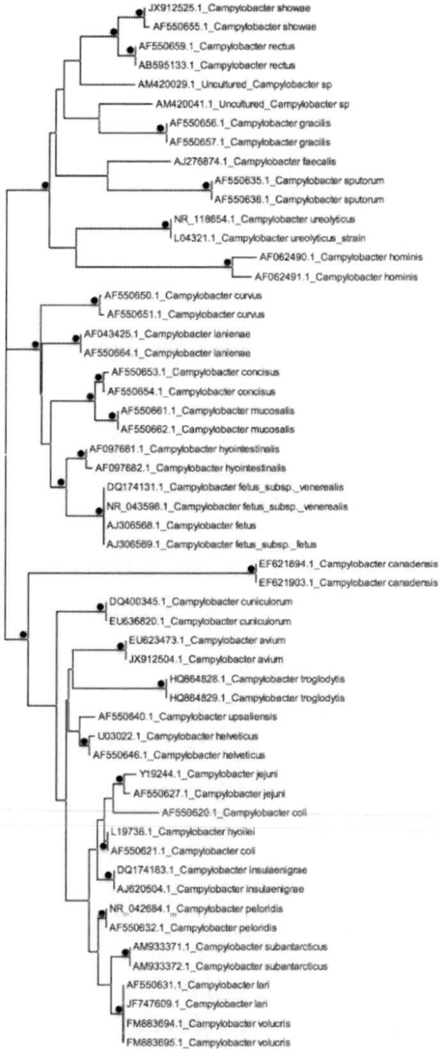

Figure 1. Evolutionary relationships of taxa . The evolutionary history of all Campylobacter species (partial 16s rRNA sequences) was inferred using the Neighbor-Joining method [59]. The optimal tree with the sum of branch length = 0.48940597 is shown. The percentage of replicate trees in which the associated taxa clustered together in the bootstrap test (100 replicates) are shown next to the branches (60). The tree is drawn to scale, with branch lengths in the same units as those of the evolutionary distances used to infer the phylogenetic tree. The evolutionary distances were computed using the Tamura-Nei method [61] and are in the units of the number of base substitutions per site. The analysis involved 55 nucleotide sequences. All positions containing gaps and missing data were eliminated. There was a total of 647 positions in the final dataset. Evolutionary analyses were conducted in MEGA5 [62].

References

[1] Nachamkin I, Blaser MJ. *Campylobacter.* 2nd Edition ed: ASM Press Washington, DC 2000.

[2] Moore JE, Corcoran D, Dooley JS, Fanning S, Lucey B, Matsuda M, McDowell DA, et al. *Campylobacter. Vet. Res.* 2005;36:351-382.

[3] Kist M. [Who discovered Campylobacter jejuni/coli? A review of hitherto disregarded literature]. *Zentralbl. Bakteriol. Mikrobiol. Hyg.* [A] 1986;261:177-186.

[4] Jones FS, Orcutt M, Little RB. Vibrios (Vibrio jejuni n. sp.) associated with intensinal disorders of cows and calves. *J. Exp. Med.* 1931;53:853-864.

[5] King EO. Human infections with Vibrio fetus and a closely related vibrio. *J. Infect Dis.* 1957;101:119-128.

[6] Skirrow MB. Campylobacter enteritis: a "new" disease. *Br. Med. J.* 1977;2:9-11.

[7] Control CfD. Outbreak of Campylobacter jejuni infections associated with drinking unpasteurized milk procured through a cow-leasing program- Wisconsin, 2001. *MMWR* 2002;51:548-549.

[8] Vogt RL, Little AA, Patton CM, Barrett TJ, Orciari LA. Serotyping and serology studies of campylobacteriosis associated with consumption of raw milk. *J. Clin. Microbiol.* 1984;20:998-1000.

[9] Control CfD. Waterborne Campylobacter gastroenteritis, Vermont. *MMWR* 1978;27:207.

[10] Grant IH, Richardson NJ, Bokkenheuser VD. Broiler chickens as potential source of Campylobacter infections in humans. *J. Clin. Microbiol.* 1980;11:508-510.

[11] Ang CW, Laman JD, Willison HJ, Wagner ER, Endtz HP, De Klerk MA, Tio-Gillen AP, et al. Structure of Campylobacter jejuni lipopolysaccharides determines antiganglioside specificity and clinical features of Guillain-Barre and Miller Fisher patients. *Infect Immun.* 2002;70:1202-1208.

[12] Fujimoto S, Allos BM, Misawa N, Patton CM, Blaser MJ. Restriction fragment length polymorphism analysis and random amplified polymorphic DNA analysis of Campylobacter jejuni strains isolated from patients with Guillain-Barre syndrome. *J. Infect Dis.* 1997;176:1105-1108.

[13] Koga M, Ang CW, Yuki N, Jacobs BC, Herbrink P, van der Meche FG, Hirata K, et al. Comparative study of preceding Campylobacter jejuni

infection in Guillain-Barre syndrome in Japan and The Netherlands. *J. Neurol. Neurosurg. Psychiatry* 2001;70:693-695.

[14] Kuroki S, Saida T, Nukina M, Haruta T, Yoshioka M, Kobayashi Y, Nakanishi H. Campylobacter jejuni strains from patients with Guillain-Barre syndrome belong mostly to Penner serogroup 19 and contain beta-N-acetylglucosamine residues. *Ann. Neurol.* 1993;33:243-247.

[15] Nachamkin I, Allos BM, Ho T. Campylobacter species and Guillain-Barre syndrome. *Clin. Microbiol. Rev.* 1998;11:555-567.

[16] Prendergast MM, Lastovica AJ, Moran AP. Lipopolysaccharides from Campylobacter jejuni O:41 strains associated with Guillain-Barre syndrome exhibit mimicry of GM1 ganglioside. *Infect Immun.* 1998;66:3649-3655.

[17] Prendergast MM, Moran AP. Lipopolysaccharides in the development of the Guillain-Barre syndrome and Miller Fisher syndrome forms of acute inflammatory peripheral neuropathies. *J. Endotoxin Res.* 2000;6:341-359.

[18] Yuki N. Infectious origins of, and molecular mimicry in, Guillain-Barre and Fisher syndromes. *Lancet Infect Dis.* 2001;1:29-37.

[19] Wassenaar TM, Newell DG. Genotyping of Campylobacter spp. *Appl. Environ. Microbiol.* 2000;66:1-9.

[20] Nachamkin I. Campylobacter infections. Current Opinion in Infectious *Diseases* 1993;6:72-76.

[21] Vandamme P, Falsen E, Pot B, Hoste B, Kersters K, De Ley J. Identification of EF group 22 campylobacters from gastroenteritis cases as Campylobacter concisus. *J. Clin. Microbiol.* 1989;27:1775-1781.

[22] Campylobacter sepsis associated with "nutritional therapy"--California. *MMWR Morb. Mortal Wkly Rep.* 1981;30:294-295

[23] Penner JL. The genus Campylobacter: a decade of progress. *Clin. Microbiol. Rev.* 1988;1:157-172.

[24] Edmonds P, Patton CM, Griffin PM, Barrett TJ, Schmid GP, Baker CN, Lambert MA, et al. Campylobacter hyointestinalis associated with human gastrointestinal disease in the United States. *J. Clin. Microbiol.* 1987;25:685-691.

[25] Gebhart CJ, Edmonds P, Ward GE, Kurtz HJ, Brenner DJ. "Campylobacter hyointestinalis" sp. nov.: a new species of Campylobacter found in the intestines of pigs and other animals. *J. Clin. Microbiol.* 1985;21:715-720.

[26] Chiu CH, Kuo CY, Ou JT. Chronic diarrhea and bacteremia caused by Campylobacter lari in a neonate. *Clin. Infect Dis.* 1995;21:700-701.

[27] Martinot M, Jaulhac B, Moog R, De Martino S, Kehrli P, Monteil H, Piemont Y. Campylobacter lari bacteremia. *Clin. Microbiol. Infect.* 2001;7:96-97.

[28] Figura N, Guglielmetti P, Zanchi A, Partini N, Armellini D, Bayeli PF, Bugnoli M, et al. Two cases of Campylobacter mucosalis enteritis in children. *J. Clin. Microbiol.* 1993;31:727-728.

[29] Soderstrom C, Schalen C, Walder M. Septicaemia caused by unusual Campylobacter species (C. laridis and C. mucosalis). *Scand. J. Infect Dis.* 1991;23:369-371.

[30] Carnahan AM, Beadling J, Watsky D, Ford N. Detection of Campylobacter upsaliensis from a blood culture by using the BacT/Alert system. *J. Clin. Microbiol.* 1994;32:2598-2599.

[31] Hanna JN, Enbom RM, Murphy DM. Campylobacter upsaliensis bacteraemia in an aboriginal child. *Med. J. Aust.* 1994;160:655-656.

[32] Gaudreau C, Lamothe F. Campylobacter upsaliensis isolated from a breast abscess. *J. Clin. Microbiol.* 1992;30:1354-1356.

[33] Chusid MJ, Wortmann DW, Dunne WM. "Campylobacter upsaliensis" sepsis in a boy with acquired hypogammaglobulinemia. *Diagn Microbiol. Infect Dis.* 1990;13:367-369.

[34] Lastovica AJ, Le Roux E, Penner JL. "Campylobacter upsaliensis" isolated from blood cultures of pediatric patients. *J. Clin. Microbiol.* 1989;27:657-659.

[35] Siqueira JF, Jr., Rocas I. A 16S rDNA-based nested PCR protocol to detect Campylobacter gracilis in oral infections. *Pesqui. Odontol. Bras.* 2003;17:142-146.

[36] Lam JY, Wu AK, Ngai DC, Teng JL, Wong ES, Lau SK, Lee RA, et al. Three cases of severe invasive infections caused by Campylobacter rectus and first report of fatal C. rectus infection. *J. Clin. Microbiol.* 2011;49:1687-1691.

[37] Mahlen SD, Clarridge JE, 3rd. Oral abscess caused by Campylobacter rectus: case report and literature review. *J. Clin. Microbiol.* 2009;47:848-851.

[38] Vandamme P, De Ley J. Proposal for a new family. Campylobacteraceae. *Int. J. Syst. Bacteriol.* 1991;41:451-455.

[39] Vandamme P, Falsen E, Rossau R, Hoste B, Segers P, Tytgat R, De Ley J. Revision of Campylobacter, Helicobacter, and Wolinella taxonomy: emendation of generic descriptions and proposal of Arcobacter gen. nov. *Int. J. Syst. Bacteriol.* 1991;41:88-103.

[40] Man SM. The clinical importance of emerging Campylobacter species. *Nat. Rev. Gastroenterol. Hepatol.* 2011;8:669-685.

[41] Nakari UM, Puhakka A, Siitonen A. Correct identification and discrimination between Campylobacter jejuni and C. coli by a standardized hippurate test and species-specific polymerase chain reaction. *Eur. J. Clin. Microbiol. Infect Dis.* 2008;27:513-518.

[42] de Saussure PP. Management of the returning traveler with diarrhea. *Therap Adv. Gastroenterol.* 2009;2:367-375.

[43] Aarestrup FM, Engberg J. Antimicrobial resistance of thermophilic Campylobacter. *Vet. Res.* 2001;32:311-321.

[44] Han J, Sahin O, Barton YW, Zhang Q. Key role of Mfd in the development of fluoroquinolone resistance in Campylobacter jejuni. *PLoS Pathog* 2008;4:e1000083.

[45] Chatzipanagiotou S, Papavasiliou E, Malamou-Lada E. Isolation of Campylobacter jejuni strains resistant to nalidixic acid and fluoroquinolones from children with diarrhea in Athens, Greece. *Eur. J. Clin. Microbiol. Infect Dis.* 1993;12:566-568.

[46] Chatzipanagiotou S, Papavasileiou E, Lakumenta A, Makri A, Nicolaou C, Chantzis K, Manganas S, et al. Antimicrobial susceptibility patterns of Campylobacter jejuni strains isolated from hospitalized children in Athens, Greece. *J. Antimicrob Chemother* 2002;49:803-805.

[47] Chatzipanagiotou S, Papavasileiou E, Lakumenta A, Makri A, Nicolaou C, Chantzis K, Manganas S, et al. Heat-stable antigen serotyping of Campylobacter jejuni strains isolated from hospitalized children in Athens, Greece. *Eur. J. Epidemiol.* 2003;18:1097-1100.

[48] Chatzipanagiotou S, Kilidireas K, Trimis G, Nicolaou C, Anagnostouli M, Athanassaki C, Giannoulia A, et al. Campylobacter jejuni O:19 serotype-associated Guillain-Barre syndrome in a child: the first case reported from Greece. *Clin. Microbiol. Infect* 2003;9:69-72.

[49] Chatzipanagiotou S, Michalopoulou M, Marinou I, Boufidou F, Papavasileiou E, Trikka-Graphakos E, Kabouri E, et al. Investigation of possible cytokine induction in peripheral blood mononuclear cells by heat-stable serotypes of Campylobacter jejuni. *Clin. Microbiol. Infect.* 2005;11:63-65.

[50] Chatzipanagiotou S, Ioannidou V, Ioannidis A, Nicolaou C, Papavasileiou E, Chaniotaki S, Vatopoulos A, et al. Absence of the plasmid-mediated quinolone resistance qnrA gene among Campylobacter jejuni clinical isolates from Greece. *Int. J. Antimicrob. Agents* 2005;26:261-262.

[51] Kordinas V, Nicolaou C, Ioannidis A, Papavasileiou E, John Legakis N, Chatzipanagiotou S. Prevalence of four virulence genes in Campylobacter jejuni determined by PCR and sequence analysis. *Mol. Diagn* 2005;9:211-215.

[52] Ioannidis A, Nicolaou C, Legakis NJ, Ioannidou V, Chatzipanagiotou S. The first database comprised of flagellin gene (flaA) types of Campylobacter jejuni human clinical isolates from Greece. *Eur. J. Epidemiol.* 2006;21:823-829.

[53] Ioannidis A, Nicolaou C, Chatzipanagiotou S. Correlation between flagellin A (flaA) genotypes and antimicrobial susceptibility patterns of Campylobacter jejuni strains isolated from children with gastroenteritis in Athens, Greece. *Mol. Diagn Ther.* 2009;13:389-395.

[54] Ioannidis A, Nicolaou C, Legakis NJ, Ioannidou V, Papavasileiou E, Voyatzi A, Chatzipanagiotou S. Genotyping of human Campylobacter jejuni isolates in Greece by pulsed-field gel electrophoresis. *Mol. Diagn Ther.* 2006;10:391-396.

[55] Ioannidou V, Ioannidis A, Magiorkinis E, Bagos P, Nicolaou C, Legakis N, Chatzipanagiotou S. Multilocus sequence typing (and phylogenetic analysis) of Campylobacter jejuni and Campylobacter coli strains isolated from clinical cases in Greece. *BMC Res. Notes* 2013;6:359.

[56] Papavasileiou E, Voyatzi A, Papavasileiou K, Makri A, Andrianopoulou I, Chatzipanagiotou S. Antimicrobial susceptibilities of Campylobacter jejuni isolates from hospitalized children in Athens, Greece, collected during 2004-2005. *Eur. J. Epidemiol.* 2007;22:77-78.

[57] Marinou I, Bersimis S, Ioannidis A, Nicolaou C, Mitroussia-Ziouva A, Legakis NJ, Chatzipanagiotou S. Identification and antimicrobial resistance of campylobacter species isolated from animal sources. *Front Microbiol.* 2012;3:58.

[58] Takkinen J, Ammon A, Robstad O, Breuer T, Campylobacter Working G. European survey on Campylobacter surveillance and diagnosis 2001. *Euro Surveill* 2003;8:207-213.

[59] Saitou N, Nei M. The neighbor-joining method: a new method for reconstructing phylogenetic trees. *Mol. Biol. Evol.* 1987;4:406-425.

[60] Felsenstein J. Confidence limits on phylogenies: An approach using the bootstrap. *Evolution* 1985;39:783-791.

[61] Tamura K, Nei M. Estimation of the number of nucleotide substitutions in the control region of mitochondrial DNA in humans and chimpanzees. *Mol. Biol. Evol.* 1993;10:512-526.

[62] Tamura K, Dudley J, Nei M, Kumar S. MEGA4: Molecular Evolutionary Genetics Analysis (MEGA) software version 4.0. *Mol. Biol. Evol.* 2007;24:1596-1599.

In: Campylobacter Infections
Editor: Brittany A. Bertucci

ISBN: 978-1-63463-858-6

Chapter 6

Control of *Campylobacter jejuni* and *Campylobacter coli* by Established and Novel Disinfectants in Poultry Processing Facilities

Amreeta Sarjit and Gary A. Dykes*
School of Science, Monash University, Jalan Lagoon Selatan, Selangor, Malaysia

Abstract

Poultry meat contaminated with *Campylobacter jejuni* and *Campylobacter coli* is a major cause of campylobacteriosis worldwide. These *Campylobacter* species are commensal organisms in the intestinal tract of live poultry and can cross contaminate carcasses during slaughter and processing. A range of chemical disinfectants are used to reduce or eliminate *Campylobacter* on poultry and in the processing environment. Organic acids, inorganic phosphates and chlorine-based disinfectants are commonly used for this purpose with varying efficiency depending on the approach taken. Temperature, pH and the concentration of the disinfectants are important parameters in determining their effectiveness

* Corresponding author email: gary.dykes@monash.edu.

and it is also essential that they do not change the organoleptic properties of the meat. Specific compounds used include lactic acid, citric acid, sodium hypochlorite, acidified sodium chlorite, benzalkonium chloride and trisodium phosphate and many of these are of potential human health concern. Novel, potentially less toxic and more environmentally friendly compounds are continually being sought to address this issue. The mode of action, effectiveness and applicability of established and novel disinfectants for the control of *Campylobacter* in poultry processing facilities are critically reviewed.

Introduction

Thermophilic campylobacters, in particular *Campylobacter jejuni* and *Campylobacter coli*, are major causes of campylobacteriosis worldwide (Keener et al., 2004; Nguyen et al., 2012; Park, 2002). These species are commensals which colonize the mucus overlying the epithelial cells of the caecum and cloaca of live poultry, and are also associated with other parts in the gastrointestinal tract, spleen and liver (Newell and Fearnley, 2003). It is suggested that the gastrointestinal tract of poultry harbors *C. jejuni* due to the binding of this species to the surface cells. Specifically, the outer membrane protein *CadF* allows them to bind to the fibronectin which connect the intestinal cells to one another (Park, 2005). During primary poultry processing bacteria may be transferred from the gastrointestinal tract, spleen and liver to the poultry meat (Newell and Fearnley, 2003). Poultry processing facilities actively implement practices to prevent cross-contamination by these pathogens.

A chicken may have as many as 10^9 viable *Campylobacter* cells per gram of content in the gastrointestinal tract (Park, 2005). Studies have also shown that turkeys and ducks are occasionally colonized by campylobacters in greater numbers than chickens (Corry and Atabay, 2001; Rosef et al., 1984). The environment in poultry processing facilities is conducive to the transfer of *Campylobacter* from infected to non-infected carcasses. This transfer is almost inevitable especially during scalding, defeathering and evisceration (Corry and Atabay, 2001; Shane, 2005). Both *C. jejuni* and *C. coli* tend to attach to poultry meat at the water-skin interface and are entrapped in the folds, crevices and pores of the meat and skin. The folds and follicles on the skin of poultry meat, and specifically that of chicken, consist of proteins, oils and possible fatty acids which enable *Campylobacter* to survive extreme cold temperatures (Lee et al., 1998). Rosequist et al. (2003) reported that incidence of campylobacteriosis can be reduced 30 times if *Campylobacter* numbers on poultry, and specifically chicken at the end of slaughter during processing, are reduced by 2 log units. Controlling numbers, rather than simply occurrence, of this pathogen on carcasses is therefore an important mechanism to prevent disease.

Effective chemical disinfectants which are economical and permitted by regulation are an important way to reduce *Campylobacter* numbers in poultry processing facilities. These disinfectants should have low levels of by-product formation and should be suitable to decontaminate carcass washers, immersion chillers, pre-chillers and other equipment used in poultry processing. Using disinfectants at concentrations certified by regulatory agencies is important in ensuring that they are not toxicogenic, mutagenic or carcinogenic. In addition, chemical disinfectants are not widely accepted in some countries due to the presence of chemical residues, discoloration of meat, sensitivity to organic material, high cost and limited effectiveness (Park et al., 2002; Riedel et al., 2009). The permitted levels of chemical disinfectants used on poultry should conform to the receiving countries poultry processing standards. Effective disinfectants should prevent cross-contamination of *Campylobacter* spp. and control the spread of *Campylobacter* spp. during poultry processing.

Table 1. Reduction of *Campylobacter* on poultry treated with acid based disinfectants

Sample	*Campylobacter* spp.	Disinfectant	Exposure time and temperature	Reduction (Log units)	References
Chicken skin and meat	*C. jejuni*	Tartaric acid	1min dip + 24 h at 5°C	3.72± 0.44	Riedel et al. (2009)
		Caprylic acid sodium salt		2.84± 0.42	
		Formic acid		>4.2	
		Lactic acid		3.87± 0.21	
Chicken wing	*C. jejuni*	Acetic acid	0.3 – 0.8 min at 4 °C	1.2-1.4	Zhao and Doyle (2006)
Chicken skin	*C.jejuni*	Lactic acid	1 min	0.8 ± 0.7	Chaine et al. (2013)

This chapter describes the effect on campylobacters of well-established compounds, such as acid based disinfectants, chlorine based disinfectants, inorganic phosphates and electrolyzed water, used in poultry processing. It also addresses the potential effectiveness of novel disinfectants, such as phytochemicals, for the control of *Campylobacter* in poultry processing facilities as this is in an area of strong current research interest. Table 1, 2 and 3 summarize studies reporting reductions of *Campylobacter* spp. on poultry meat treated with acid based disinfectants, chlorine based disinfectants and other types of chemical based disinfectants. All types of chemical based disinfectants reduced *Campylobacter* (~0.8-3.7 log units) on different chicken parts at different exposure times and temperatures. Although research has been reported on the use of disinfectants to reduce *Campylobacter* in chicken juice or broth, we have focused primarily on work addressing *Campylobacter* on poultry meat. Studies performed on meat are likely to produce different results as compared to studies conducted in chicken juices or broths. The poultry meat matrix could conceivably ameliorate the effect of disinfectants through, for example, buffering effects.

Colonization and Contamination of Poultry by *C. jejuni* and *C. coli*

Campylobacter is usually not detectable in broiler chickens less than 2-3 weeks old under commercial production conditions (Annan-Prah and Janc, 1988; Berndtson et al., 1996; Evans and Sayers, 2000; Jacobs-Reitsma et al., 1995; Shreeve et al., 2000; Stern et al., 2001). Studies have shown that *C. jejuni* specific maternal antibodies are present in egg yolk and the sera of 1 week old chicks and contribute to complement-mediated killing of some *C. jejuni* strains *in vitro* (Sahin et al., 2001). Other factors contributing towards *Campylobacter* being undetectable in young birds are intestinal development and the nature of the microbial flora of poultry less than 3 weeks old (Sahin et al., 2002). Poultry in commercial operations are colonized by campylobacters from 3 to 4 weeks old (Corry and Atabay, 2001; Humphrey et al., 1993; Kapperud et al., 1993; Sahin et al., 2002).

There are two modes of transmission of *Campylobacter* spp. with respect to poultry, namely horizontal and vertical transmission. Horizontal transmission is the most common and widely established mode of infection of poultry by *Campylobacter* spp. from the environment while vertical transmission is regarded as relatively rare (Altekruse et al., 1999; Sahin et al., 2002). Various molecular epidemiological studies conducted on grandparent flocks positive for *Campylobacter* spp. have not been able to show vertical transmission into parent flocks (Callicott et al., 2006). Sources of horizontal transmission include contaminated water, litter, insects, wild birds, rodents, fecal-oral contact, and farm and poultry processing personnel (Aarts et al., 1995; Evan and Sayers, 2000; Line, 2001). In addition, chickens are coprophagic which enhances the dissemination of *Campylobacter* spp. among poultry flocks (Park, 2005).

Thermophilic campylobacters, such as *C. jejuni* and *C. coli,* are fastidious and not able to grow outside their host in the environment but their ability to attach to poultry and poultry processing surfaces is well established. Contamination of poultry meat by *Campylobacter* can be affected by factors related to the host and by environmental conditions associated with the processing line. As indicated above, colonization by *C. jejuni* and *C. coli* occurs in the gastrointestinal tract of poultry and these species must therefore be able to withstand the stresses, such as pH and bile, imposed by this environment (Park, 2005). Thermophilic campylobacters have an optimal growth temperature of 37 to 42°C (Altekruse et al., 1999) and the temperature at which they grow may influence their subsequent survival. For example, Duffy and Dykes (2006) reported that *C. jejuni* grown at 37°C, which is the body temperature of humans, are better able to survive in water at 4°C than those grown at 42°C, which is the temperature of avian gut.

The spread of *C. jejuni* and *C. coli* can occur by carry-over of *Campylobacter* spp. from a positive flock to a new flock. It should be noted that once a flock becomes infected with *C. jejuni* and *C. coli*, cells can multiply and spread rapidly to most of the birds within the flock and persist until slaughter, leading to carcass contamination during poultry processing (Sahin et al., 2002). Crates used to transport poultry to the abattoir can also cause this carry-over and act as a source of contamination. The genotypes of strains vary substantially indicating that a single source of *Campylobacter* transmission from farm to processing level is unlikely (Sahin et al., 2002).

The skin on the chicken meat is usually not removed during processing and this surface may allow the attachment of *Campylobacter* originating from intestinal contents, feces or contaminated equipment (Corry and Atabay, 2001). *Campylobacter* adheres to the skin surface by both physiochemical and receptor specific mechanisms making them difficult to remove with water (Corry and Atabay, 2001). Carcass rinsing with water will immediately remove some *Campylobacter* contamination but because of the uptake of water by the carcass some *Campylobacter* cells are trapped in the folds and crevices of the skin (Corry and Atabay, 2001).

Acid Based Disinfectants

Studies have shown that *Campylobacter* are unable to survive at low pH (4.0 and 4.5) while their optimum pH for survival is from 6.5 to 7.5 (Shaheen et al., 2007). Treating these pathogens with acids, and specifically organic acids, many of which are regarded as safe for human consumption, is a widely applied control.

Organic acids, such as lactic acid, are natural compounds produced during postmortem glycolysis in meat and have minimal effects on the organoleptic effects of meat at low concentration and when produced under these conditions (Goncalves et al., 2005). Studies have shown that the bactericidal mode of action of lactic acid and other organic acids is due to the lowering of pH which impairs the ability of *Campylobacter* cells to survive on meat. The undissociated acid molecules in organic acids that penetrate the membrane of *Campylobacter* cells lead to metabolic inhibition and acidification of the cytoplasm (Booth, 1985; Birk et al., 2010; Vasseur et al., 1999). Organic acids that have been found to be effective in reducing *C. jejuni* on poultry, specifically chicken meat, include acetic acid, lactic acid and tartaric acid among others (Table 1). These disinfectants reduce *C. jejuni* (~0.8-3.7 log units) on different chicken parts at different exposure times and temperatures. Of the acids listed tartaric acid resulted in the highest log reduction of *C. jejuni* on chicken skin and meat, while lactic acid resulted in the lowest log reduction of *C. jejuni* on chicken skin. Differences in the nature of the acids, such as their pKa, as well as exposure times and the food matrix may have resulted in differences in reduction of numbers of *C. jejuni* on chicken in the studies listed.

The concentration of an acid and pH of the solution used in poultry processing facilities is important in ensuring that it does not damage the poultry meat and is not corrosive to the equipment. These two parameters also play a role in determining the number of viable *Campylobacter* cells after treatment with an acid. Treatment with an effective concentration of organic acid at low pH can sometimes result in the discoloration of meat. This can be prevented by using buffered lactic (or other) acid as their mode of action has been shown to be related to undissociated acid molecules rather than the pH of the solution (Bolder, 1997).

Differences in the meat matrix of poultry will influence the effects of organic acids on *Campylobacter* during acid stress. The buffering capacity of the meat and the diminished accessibility of organic acids to *Campylobacter* enables its survival on meat. Studies indicate that after adding an organic acid with a low pH onto the meat surface there was an increase in pH within a few minutes which neutralized the antibacterial effect resulting in protection of the bacterial cells (Birk et al., 2010).

Campylobacter strains are more sensitive to organic acids if the temperature is raised. Citric acid was found to be more effective at 50°C compared to 4°C or 20°C because acid dissociation constants are inversely affected by temperature. Treatments are also more effective at a higher temperature due to the changes in the fatty acid content of the bacterial membrane and removal of *Campylobacter* cells from the skin caused by the softening of fat and lowering of surface tension (Alonso-Hernando et al., 2013). Concerns have been raised that the natural acid resistance of each strain and methodology used for acid adaptation, such as pH adjustment, may lead to survival of *Campylobacter* on meat (Samelis, 2005)

Chlorine Based Disinfectants

Chlorine based disinfectants have been used in poultry processing for more than four decades to reduce cross-contamination of pathogens on meat and equipment surfaces (Bashor et al., 2004). The efficacy of chlorine in reducing *Campylobacter* decreases with increasing pH. When using chlorine based disinfectants it is important to ensure that the concentration of chlorine used produces free residuals. To ensure antimicrobial efficacy is at its peak, a free residual chlorine at a low temperature and between pH 4 to 6 is used since chlorine is completely hydrolyzed to hypochlorous acid (HOCl) under these conditions when it is mixed with water (Bashor et al., 2004). The presence of hypochlorous acid causes denaturation of protein by oxidation, enzyme inhibition and disruption of the cell wall leading to cell death (Morato et al., 2003). The concentration of the residual chlorine, which is proportional to the rate of *Campylobacter* inactivation and the pH of water after the addition of chlorine, is important in determining the reduction of *Campylobacter* (Keener et al., 2004). Organic load also influences the effect of chlorine as chlorine binds to the organic matter present. It is therefore important that organic matter is consistently and effectively removed from poultry washers to maintain the activity of chlorine (Bashor et al., 2004). Chlorine based disinfectants have been shown to reduce *Campylobacter* on poultry, specifically chicken meat, as shown in Table 2. These disinfectants reduced *C. jejuni* (~2.1-3.7 log units) on different chicken parts at different exposure time and temperatures. Of the chlorine based disinfectants listed, chlorhexidine diacetate salt hydrate resulted in the highest log reduction of *C. jejuni* on chicken skin and meat while sodium hypochlorite resulted in the lowest log reduction of *Campylobacter* spp. on chicken carcass. An exposure time of one minute to some disinfectants was sufficient to result in a reduction in *Campylobacter* numbers even after 24 hours of cold storage (Table 2).

Table 2. Reduction of *Campylobacter* on poultry treated with chlorine based disinfectants

Sample	*Campylobacter* spp.	Disinfectant	Exposure time and temperature	Reduction (Log units)	References
Chicken skin and meat	*C. jejuni*	Chlorhexidine diacetate salt hydrate	1min dip + 24 h at 5°C	3.70± 0.49	Riedel et al. (2009)
		Cetylpyridinium chloride		2.26± 0.91	
		Benzalkonium chloride		3.38± 0.58	
Chicken carcass	*Campylobacter* spp.	Sodium hypochlorite	15 s	~2.1	Northcutt et al. (2007)
Chicken carcass	*C. jejuni*	Acidified sodium chlorite at an adjusted pH 2.5-2.6 using citric acid	20 s at 25 °C	>3 log	Sexton et al. (2007)
Chicken carcass	*Campylobacter* spp.	Acidified sodium chlorite	0.3 min at 14 - 18 °C	2.6	Kemp et al. (2001)

Hypochlorite (HOCl) is commonly used as a chlorine-based disinfectant due to the fact that it rapidly forms hypochlorous acid when mixed with water. Sodium hypochlorite, a common hypochlorite used in poultry processing facilities, is effective in decreasing or killing pathogens when the pH is lower than 7.5 (Gavin and Weddig, 1995). Hypochlorite is known to inhibit glucose oxidation by the chlorine-oxidizing sulfhydryl groups of certain enzymes important in carbohydrate metabolism (Huang et al., 2007).

Chlorine dioxide (ClO_2) is another disinfectant which has been used for many decades. This chlorine based disinfectant does not, however, form hypochlorous acid when mixed with water. It has no association with pH and is used at much lower concentration unlike other chlorine disinfectants (Keener et al., 2004). The mode of action of chlorine dioxide is to disrupt the transport of nutrients across the cell wall and is usually used in amounts not exceeding 3 ppm residual chlorine dioxide in poultry processing chiller water. Chlorine dioxide does not affect the organoleptic quality of meat but tends to cause a slight discoloration on meat. To our knowledge, the action of chlorine dioxide against *C. jejuni* or *C. coli* specifically during poultry processing has yet to be investigated.

Acidified sodium chlorite (ASC) is used as a disinfectant during poultry processing and is produced with a food grade acid, such as citric acid, and sodium chlorite. Chlorous acid is formed immediately due to the chemical reaction between acid and chlorite. The ideal pH for ASC is between 2.3 to 3.2 at ambient temperature when it is able to oxidize the microbial cell wall, disrupting the sulfide and disulfide linkage of protein leading to the disruption of the amino acid component of the cell membrane (Keener et al., 2004).

Chlorine based disinfectants are effective for inactivation of *Campylobacter* in biofilms (of other bacterial species) as it completely inactivates *C. jejuni* in biofilms after treatment at a concentration of 50 ppm for 45 seconds (Alter and Scherer, 2006). *C. jejuni* is sensitive to conditions outside the host, suggesting that it has a low possibility of being a primary colonizer for biofilm formation in the environment (Teh et al., 2014). Studies have suggested that *C. jejuni* can act as a secondary colonizer of well-established biofilms of other bacterial species instead, resulting in a multispecies biofilm (Hanning et al., 2008). In addition, *C. jejuni* is able to survive in a multispecies biofilm under conditions that do not usually permit its growth as they depend on the uptake of secondary metabolites such as carbon or energy sources produced by other bacteria present in the multispecies biofilm (Pearson et al., 1993; Teh et al., 2014; Trachoo et al., 2002).

Inorganic Phosphates

Trisodium phosphate (TSP) is a well known inorganic phosphate which has been used as an antimicrobial in poultry washers (Capita et al., 2002). It is generally used at concentrations between 8 to 12% which renders no negative effects on the organoleptic quality of meat. This compound is used in chiller water at pH 10 to 12 and has a destructive effect on bacteria. Gram negative bacteria are much more susceptible to alkaline sanitizers, such as TSP, at high pH than Gram positive bacteria because of their thin peptidoglycan layer (Capita et al., 2002; Dickson et al., 1994; Sampathkumar et al., 2003). High pH weakens the cells ability to prevent the cytoplasmic membrane from bursting (Mendonca et al., 1994). The antimicrobial properties of TSP are also due to complex linkage formation with bivalent metals which in turn interferes with the cell wall stability of the microorganism (Luck and Jager, 1997;

Pohlman et al., 2002). Due to its surfactant properties TSP may aid in the removal of *Campylobacter* that have not firmly attached to the skin of poultry. It also causes the removal of some surface fat and this aids in the reduction of *Campylobacter* during the washing process. TSP has the ability to remove the protective lipid layer on meat to reach the follicles where *Campylobacter* is entrapped resulting in the reduction of this pathogen on meat (Capita et al., 2002). The role of TSP in the reduction of *Campylobacter* spp. on poultry, specifically chicken meat, has been well studied as shown in Table 3. It has been shown to reduce *C. jejuni* (~1.5-3.7 log units) on chicken skin with meat and chicken carcass at different exposure times and temperatures. An increased TSP exposure time on poultry may not necessarily result in a higher reduction of *Campylobacter* spp. on meat. Poultry production facilities usually prefer a shorter decontamination treatment time which is more feasible for application in their in-line operations during processing (Riedel et al., 2009).

Table 3. Reduction of *Campylobacter* on poultry treated with chemical disinfectants

Sample	*Campylobacter* spp.	Disinfectant	Exposure time and temperature	Reduction (Log units)	References
Chicken skin and meat	*C. jejuni*	Trisodium phosphate	1min dip + 24 h at 5°C	3.69± 0.27	Riedel et al. (2009)
Chicken carcass	*Campylobacter* spp.	Trisodium phosphate	50 °C + 24 h	1.5	Slavik et al. (1994)
Chicken carcass (neck skin)	*Campylobacter* spp.	Trisodium phosphate	15 s	1.7	Whyte et al. (2001)
Chicken wings	*C. jejuni*	Electrolyzed water containing 50 mg/L residual chlorine	10 min at 4 °C 30 min at 4 °C 10 min at 23 °C 30 min at 23 °C	3	Park et al. (2002)
Chicken meat	*C.jejuni*	Rosemary extract (V40)	1min dip + 48 h and pre-freezing	>2	Piskernik et al. (2011)

Electrolyzed Oxidizing Water

Electrolyzed oxidizing water (EO) is gaining popularity as an antimicrobial on food and its processing surfaces (Huang et al., 2007; Hricova et al., 2008). It is formed by electrolyzing a sodium chloride solution into a basic and acidic fraction. The basic fraction has a pH of about 11 and is formed at the cathode, and the acidic fraction has a pH of about 2.6 and is formed at the anode (Kim et al., 2005). Although it has a strong acid present, it is non corrosive to the skin of the poultry meat due to the transfer of ions from the anode to cathode. This disinfectant represents a non-thermal approach to inactivate *Campylobacter* and only requires a very dilute salt solution to generate the EO (Park et al., 2002). EO also prevents cross-contamination and poses less potential hazard to poultry processing personnel handling concentrated chemicals (Park et al., 2002). The disadvantage of using EO, however, is the need to continuously supply hypochlorite and chlorine by electrolysis to sustain the antimicrobial effect (Kiura et al., 2002).

EO has been used to reduce *C. jejuni* on chicken wings as shown in Table 3 (Park et al., 2002). The duration of exposure and temperature did not affect the reduction of the bacterial load attached to the meat. Electrolyzed water is known to rapidly kill *Campylobacter* located at water-skin interfaces as the EO penetrates into the crevices or pores that protect *Campylobacter*. In addition, its mode of action is associated with the presence of hypochlorous acid, high oxidation reduction potential and low pH (Park et al., 2002). The presence of hypochlorous acid inactivates *Campylobacter* cells via oxidation of cell surface sulfhydryl compounds and inactivation enzymes involved in respiration and inhibition of ATP generation (Park et al., 2002). It has been suggested that EO has a similar effect to TSP with respect to removing fat and killing bacterial cells on the surface of chicken skin (Capita et al., 2002).

Novel Compounds As Alternatives to Current Disinfectants

There is a growing interest in using natural bioactive compounds to reduce *Campylobacter* in poultry processing facilities. Current established disinfectants, if used excessively, may eventually lead to increased adaptation of *Campylobacter* to stressful environments and this acquisition of resistance may enhance its survival on poultry meat (Langsrud et al., 2003). Natural bioactive compounds may also be better accepted by consumers since they are safe and natural occurring compounds (Lopez-Malo et al., 2005; Piskernik et al., 2011). Their use may also help reduce the oxidative degradation of lipids and proteins which in turn improves the quality of meat. Studies have shown that naturally occurring compounds such as epigallocatechin gallate (EGCG), chlorogenic acid, gallic acid, sinapinic acid, vanillic acid, syringic acid, ferrulic acid, rosmanic acid and carnosic acid possess antimicrobial activity against *C. jejuni* and *C. coli* (Klancnik et al., 2012; Sarjit et al., 2014).

Rosemary extract (*Rosmarinus officinalis L.*) is used as a functional food and its extract formulations, such as V40, containing rosmarinic and carnosic acid have anti-*Campylobacter* activity as shown in Table 3 (Piskernik et al., 2011). The mode of action of this extract against *Campylobacter* is associated with the absence of a stress adaptive response but the exact mechanism behind this stress sensitivity needs to be further investigated (Klancnik et al., 2012).

Gallic acid has antimicrobial activity against *C. jejuni* and *C. coli*. The mode of action of this bioactive phytochemical is not only caused by the low pH of the medium but also by the loss of calcium ions in *C. coli* specifically, due to the impairment of the permeability of cellular membranes (Sarjit et al., 2014).

These naturally occurring compounds may be potential antimicrobials that can be used to control *Campylobacter* in a poultry processing facility. However, further studies need to be done to elucidate the exact mechanisms and optimized parameters to be used in a poultry processing facility. One of the drawbacks in using naturally occurring compounds is it may affect the organoleptic qualities of poultry meat. Studies have found that dietary garlic supplements changes the color, taste and smell of the meat (Cross et al., 2011). In addition naturally occurring compounds used as potential antimicrobials should not result in lower effectiveness, higher cost or product organoleptic quality deterioration. Further research needs to be conducted on the development of purification procedures of active compounds which will also reduce the loss of functional properties of these compounds (Negi et al., 2012).

Conclusion

Many of the interventions described above have the potential to be used to control the cross contamination of *C. jejuni* and *C. coli* during poultry processing. Many of the studies described above demonstrating activity of compounds against *Campylobacter* have been carried out in the laboratory. It is important to perform these studies at pilot or industrial sites to mimic commercial conditions and validate the results obtained before conclusions on their efficacy can be drawn. In addition there are few detailed studies establishing the mode of action and optimized parameters for many of these compounds used. Further studies need to be conducted to elucidate these so that they can be effectively applied and controlled. In addition, the levels of residues of each compound on poultry meat should be tested to ensure there are no health concerns for consumers. Many countries are involved in the production of other types of poultry such as duck and turkey in addition to chicken meat. Further studies on the use of control measures on all types of poultry are required to confirm they are effective in controlling *Campylobacter* on different products.

Reduction in numbers of *C. jejuni* and *C. coli* may be achieved by incorporating chemical based disinfectants at different stages during poultry processing. This should in turn result in reduced campylobacteriosis in the population and improve public health outcomes (Rosequist et al., 2003). These will be enhanced if rational harmonized regulations and standards for poultry at an international level are established. Interactions between industry, research and academic institutions are important to generate and publish data. This communication will be invaluable in reducing *Campylobacter* and campylobacteriosis associated with poultry.

References

Aarts, H.J., van Lith, L.A. & Jacobs-Reitsma, W.F. (1995). Discrepancy between Penner serotyping and polymerase chain reaction fingerprinting of *Campylobacter* isolated from poultry and other animal sources. *Letters in Applied Microbiology,* 20, 371-374.

Alonso-Hernando, A., Guevara-Franco, J.A., Alonso-Calleja, C. & Capita, R. (2013). Effect of the temperature of dipping solution on the antimicrobial effectiveness of various chemical decontaminants against pathogenic and spoilage bacteria on poultry. *Journal of Food Protection,* 76, 833-842.

Alter, T. & Scherer, K. (2006). Stress response of *Campylobacter* spp. and its role in food processing. *Journal of Veterinary Medicine Series* B, 53, 351–357.

Altekruse, S. F., Stern, N. J., Fields, P. I. & Swerdlow, D. L. (1999). *Campylobacter jejuni*-an emerging foodborne pathogen. *Emerging Infectious Disease,* 5, 28-35.

Annan-Prah, A. & Janc, M. (1988). The mode of spread of *Campylobacter jejuni/coli* to broiler flocks. *Journal of Veterinary Medicine B*, 35, 11-18.

Bashor, M.P., Curtis, P.A., Keener, K.M., Sheldon, B.W., Kathariou, S. & Osbornes, J.A. (2004). Effect of carcass washers on *Campylobacter* contamination in large broiler processing plants. *Poultry Science,* 83, 1232-1239.

Berndtson, E., Danielsson-Tham, M-L. & Engvall, A. (1996). *Campylobacter* incidence on a chicken farm and the spread of *Campylobacter* during the slaughter process. *International Journal of Food Microbiology,* 32, 35-47.

Birk, T., Gronlund, A.C., Christensen, B.B., Knochel, S., Lohse, K. & Rosequist, H. (2010). Effect of organic acids and marination ingredients on the survival of *Campylobacter jejuni* on meat. *Journal of Food Protection,* 73, 258-265.

Bolder, N. (1997). Decontamination of meat and poultry carcasses. *Food Science Technology*, 5, 384 – 389.

Booth, I. R.(1985). Regulation of cytoplasmic pH in bacteria. *Microbiological Reviews,* 49, 359–37.

Callicott, K.A., Fridhriksdóttir, V., Reiersen, J., Lowman, R., Bisaillon, J., Gunnarsson, E., Berndtson, E., Hiett, K.L., Needleman, D.S. & Stern, N.J. (2006). Lack of evidence for vertical transmission of *Campylobacter* spp. in chickens. *Applied and Environmental Microbiology*, 72, 5794–5798.

Capita, R., Alonso-Calleja, C., García-Fernández, M.C. & Moreno, B. (2002). Review: trisodium phosphate treatment for decontamination of poultry. *Food Science and Technology International,* 8, 11-24.

Chaine, A., Arnaud, E., Kondjoyan, A., Collignan, A. & Sarter, S. (2013). Effect of steam and lactic acid treatments on the survival of *Salmonella* Enteritidis and *Campylobacter jejuni* inoculated on chicken skin. *International Journal of Food Microbiology,* 162, 276-282.

Corry, J.E.L. & Atabay, H.I. (2001). Poultry as a source of *Campylobacter* and related organisms. *Journal of Applied Microbiology,* 90, 96S-114S.

Cross, D.E., McDevitt, R.M. & Acamovic, T. (2011). Herbs, thyme essential oil and condensed tannin extracts as dietary supplements for broilers, and their effects on performance, digestibility, volatile fatty acids and organoleptic properties. *British Poultry Science*, 52, 227-237.

Dickson, J.S., Nettles Cutter, C.G. & Siragusa, G.R. (1994). Antimicrobial effects of trisodium phosphate against bacteria attached to beef tissue. *Journal of Food Protection,* 57, 952-955.

Duffy, L. & Dykes, G.A. (2006). Growth temperatures of four *Campylobacter jejuni* strains influence their subsequent survival in food and water. *Letters in Applied Microbiology*, 43, 596-601.

Evans, S.J. & Sayers, A.R. (2000). A longitudinal study of *Campylobacter* infection of broiler flocks in Great Britain. *Preventive Veterinary Medicine,* 46, 209-223.

Gavin, A. & Weddig, L.M. (1995). *Canned foods: Principles of Thermal Process Control, Acidification and Container Closure Evaluation* (6th ed). Washington, D.C: The Food Processors Institute.

Gonçalves, A.C., Almeida, R.C.C., Alves, M.A.O. & Almeida, P.F. (2005). Quantitative investigation of the effects of chemical treatments in reducing *Listeria monocytogenes* populations on chicken breast meat. *Food Control*, 16, 617–622.

Hanning, I., Jarquin, R. & Slavik, M. (2008). *Campylobacter jejuni* as a secondary colonizer of poultry biofilms. *Journal of Applied Microbiology,* 105, 1199-1208.

Hricova, D., Stephan, R. & Zweifel, C. (2008). Electrolyzed water and its application in the food industry. *Journal of Food Protection,* 71, 1934–1947.

Huang, Y.R., Hung Y.C., Hsu, S.Y., Huang, Y.W. & Hwang, D.F. (2007). Application of electrolyzed water in the food industry. *Food Control*, 19, 329-345.

Humphrey, T.J., Henley, A. & Lanning, D.G. (1993). The colonization of broiler chickens with *Campylobacter jejuni*: some epidemiological investigations. *Epidemiology and Infection,* 110, 601-607.

Jacobs-Reitsma, W.F., van der Giessen, A.W., Bolder, N.M. & Mulder, R.W.A.W. (1995). Epidemiology of *Campylobacter* spp. at two Dutch broiler farms. *Epidemiology and Infection,* 114, 413-421.

Kapperud, G., Skjerve, E., Vik, L., Hauge, K., Lysaker, A., Aalmen, I., Ostroff, S.M. &

Potter, M. (1993). Epidemiological investigation of risk factors for *Campylobacter* colonization in Norwegian broiler flocks. *Epidemiological Infection,* 111, 245-255.

Kemp, G. K., Aldrich, M. L., Guerra, M. L. & Schneider, K. R. (2001). Continuous online processing of fecal-and ingesta-contaminated poultry carcasses using an acidified sodium chlorite antimicrobial intervention. *Journal of Food Protection,* 64, 807–812.

Keener, K.M., Bashor, M.P., Curtis, P.A., Sheldon, B.W. & Kathariou, S. (2004). Comprehensive review of *Campylobacter* and poultry processing. *Comprehensive Reviews in Food Science and Food Safety,* 3, 105–116.

Kim, C., Hung, Y.C. & Russell, S.M. (2005). Efficacy of electrolyzed water in the prevention and removal of fecal material attachment and its microbicidal effectiveness. *Poultry Science,* 84, 1778-1784.

Kiura, H., Sano, K., Morimatsu, S., Nakano, T., Morita, C., Yamaguchi, M., Maeda, T. & Katsuoka, Y. (2002). Bactericidal activity of electrolyzed acid water from solution containing sodium chloride at low concentration, in comparison with that at high concentration. *International Journal of Food Microbiology Methods,* 49, 285–293.

Klancnik, A., Mozina, S.S. & Zhang, Q. (2012). Anti- *Campylobacter* activities and resistance mechanisms of natural phenolic compounds in *Campylobacter. PLoS ONE,* 7, e51800.

Langsrud, S., Sidhu, M.S., Heir, E. & Holck, A.L. (2003). Bacterial disinfectant resistance-a challenge for the food industry. *International Biodeterioration and Biodegradation,* 51, 283-290.

Lee, A., Smith, S.C. & Coloe, P.J. (1998). Survival and growth of *Campylobacter jejuni* after artificial inoculation onto chicken skin as a function of temperature and packaging conditions. *Journal of Food Protection,* 61, 1609–1614.

Line, J.E. (2001). *Campylobacter* and *Salmonella* levels for poultry raised on litter. *Poultry Science,* 81, 1473-1481.

Lopez-Malo, A., Alzamora, S.M. & Palou, E. (2005). *Naturally Occurring Compounds: Plant Sources. In*: Davidson, P.M., Sofos, J.N., Branen, A.L., (3rd ed), Antimicrobials in Food (ed, pp 429-452). New York: CRC Press.

Luck, E. & Jager, M. (1997). *Antimicrobial food additives, characteristics, uses, effects.* (2nd ed). Berlin: Springer-Verlag.

Morato, J., Mir, J., Codony, F., Mas, J. & Ribas, F. (2003). Microbial response to disinfectants. In: Mara, D. Horan, N. (ed.), *The Handbook of Water and Wastewater Microbiology* (pp 657-693). London: Elsevier.

Mendonca, A.F., Amoroso, T.L. & Knabel, S.J. (1994). Destruction of gram-negative foodborne pathogens by high pH involves disruption of the cytoplasmatic membrane. *Applied and Environmental Microbiology,* 60, 4009-4014.

Negi, P.S. (2012). Plant extracts for the control of bacterial growth: Efficacy, stability and safety issues for food application. *International Journal of Food Microbiology,* 156, 7-17.

Newell, D.G. & Fearnley, C. (2003). Sources of *Campylobacter* colonization in broiler chickens. *Applied and Environmental Microbiology,* 69, 4343-4351.

Nguyen, V.T., Fegan, N., Turner, M.S. & Dykes, G.A. (2012). Role of attachment to surfaces on the prevalence and survival of *Campylobacter* through food systems. *Journal of Food Protection,* 75, 195-206.

Northcutt, J., Smith, D., Ingram, K.D., Hinton Jr, A. & Musgrove, M. (2007). Recovery of bacteria from broiler carcasses after spray washing with acidified electrolyzed water or sodium hypochlorite solutions. *Poultry Science,* 86, 2239–2244.

Park, H., Hung, Y.C. & Brackett, R.E. (2002). Antimicrobial effect of electrolyzed water for inactivating *Campylobacter jejuni* during poultry washing. *International Journal of Food Microbiology,* 72, 77-83.

Park, S.F. (2005). *Campylobacter jejuni* stress responses during survival in the food chain and colonization In Ketley, J.M., Konkel, M.E. (Eds), *Campylobacter : Molecular and Cellular Biology* (ed, pp. 311) Great Britain: Horizon Bioscience.

Pearson, A.D., Greenwood, M., Healing, T. D., Rollins, D., Shahamat, M., Donaldson, J. & Colwell, R.R. (1993). Colonization of broiler chickens by waterborne *Campylobacter jejuni. Applied and Environmental Microbiology, 59,* 987-996.

Piskernik, S., Klancnik, A., Riedel, C.T., Brondsted, L. & Mozina, S.S. (2011).

Reduction of *Campylobacter jejuni* by natural antimicrobials in chicken meat-related conditions. *Food Control,* 22, 718-724.

Pohlman, F.W., Stivarius, M.R., McElyea, K.S. & Waldroup, A.L. (2002). Reduction of *E.coli, Salmonella typhimurium*, coliforms, aerobic bacteria and improvement of ground beef color using trisodium phosphate or cetylpyridinium chloride before grinding. *Meat Science,* 60, 349–356.

Riedel, C. T., Brøndsted, L., Rosenquist, H., Haxgart, S. N. & Christensen, B. B. (2009). Chemical decontamination of *Campylobacter jejuni* on chicken skin and meat. *Journal of Food Protection,* 72, 1173–1180.

Rosef, O., Gondrosen, B. & Kapperud, G. (1984). *Campylobacter jejuni* and *Campylobacter coli* as surface contaminants of fresh and frozen poultry carcasses. *International Journal Food Microbiology,* 1, 205–215.

Rosenquist, H., Nielsen, N.L., Sommer, H.M., Nørrung, B. & Christensen, B.B. (2003). Quantitative risk assessment of human campylobacteriosis associated with thermotolerant *Campylobacter* species in chickens. *International Journal of Food Microbiology,* 83, 87–103.

Sahin, O., Morishita, T.Y. & Zhang, Q. (2002). *Campylobacter* colonization in poultry: sources of infection and modes of transmission. *Animal Health Research Reviews,* 3, 95-105.

Sahin, O., Zhang, Q. & Meitzler, J.C. (2001). Effect of anti-*Campylobacter* maternal antibody on the colonization of *C.jejuni* in poultry. *Proceeding of the American Society for Microbiology,* 101st General Meeting, Orlando, Florida, USA, pp742-743.

Samelis, J. (2005). Meat decontamination and pathogen stress adaptation. In J. N. Sofos (Ed.), *Improving the safety of fresh meat* (pp. 562–591). Cambridge, England: Woodhead Publishing Limited.

Sampathkumar, B., Khachatourians, G.G. & Korber, D.R. (2003). High pH during trisodium phosphate treatment causes membrane damage and destruction of *Salmonella* enterica Serovar Enteritidis. *Applied and Environmental Microbiology, 69*, 122-129.

Sarjit, A., Wang, Y. & Dykes, G.A. (2014). Antimicrobial activity of gallic acid against thermophilic *Campylobacter* is strain specific and associated with a loss of calcium ions. *Food Microbiology,* 46, 227-233.

Sexton, M., Raven, G., Holds, G., Pointon, A., Kiermeier, A. & Sumner, J. (2007). Effect of acidified sodium chlorite treatment on chicken carcasses processed in South Australia. *International Journal of Food Microbiology,* 115, 252-255.

Shaheen, B.W., Miller, M.E. & Oyarzabal, O.A. (2007). *In vitro* survival at low pH and acid adaptation response of *Campylobacter jejuni* and *Campylobacter coli. Food Safety,* 27, 326-343.

Shane, S. (2005). *Handbook on poultry diseases.* (2nd ed). Singapore, American Soybean Association.

Shreeve, J.E., Toszeghy, M., Pattison, M. & Newell, D.G. (2000). Sequential spread of *Campylobacter* infection in a multi-pen broiler house. *Avian Disease,* 44, 983-988.

Slavik, M. F., Kim, J.W., Pharr, M. D., Raben, D. P., Tsai, S. & Lobsinger, C. M. (1994). Effect of trisodium phosphate on *Campylobacter* attached to post-chill chicken carcasses. *Journal of Food Protection,* 57, 324–326.

Stern, N.J., Fedorka-Cray, P., Bailey, J.S., Cox, N.A., Craven, S.E., Hiett, K.L., Musgrove, M.T., Ladely, S., Cosby, D. & Mead, G.C. (2001). Distribution of *Campylobacter* spp. in selected U.S. poultry production and processing operations. *Journal of Food Protection,* 64, 1705-1710.

Teh, A.H.T., Lee, S.M. & Dykes, G.A. (2014). Does *Campylobacter jejuni* form biofilms in food related environments? *Applied and Environmental Microbiology,* 80, 5154-5160.

Trachoo, N., Frank, J.F. & Stern, N.J. (2002). Survival of *Campylobacter jejuni* in biofilms isolated from chicken houses. *Journal of Food Protection,* 65, 1110-1116.

Vasseur, C., Baverel, L., Hebraud, M. & Labadie, J. (1999). Effect of osmotic, alkaline, acid or thermal stresses on the growth and inhibition of *Listeria monocytogenes*. *Journal of Applied Microbiology*, 86, 469–476.

Whyte, P., Collins, J.D., McGill, K., Monahan, C. & O' Mahony, H. (2001). Quantitative investigation of the effects of chemical decontamination procedures on the microbiological status of broiler carcasses during processing. *Journal of Food Protection,* 64, 179-183.

Zhao, T. & Doyle, M. P. (2006). Reduction of *Campylobacter jejuni* on chicken wings by chemical treatments. *Journal of Food Protection,* 69, 762–767.

Index

C

D

E

F

I

J

K

L

M

N

O

P

Q

R

S